The Pharmacy Technician Series

PHARMACY CALCULATIONS

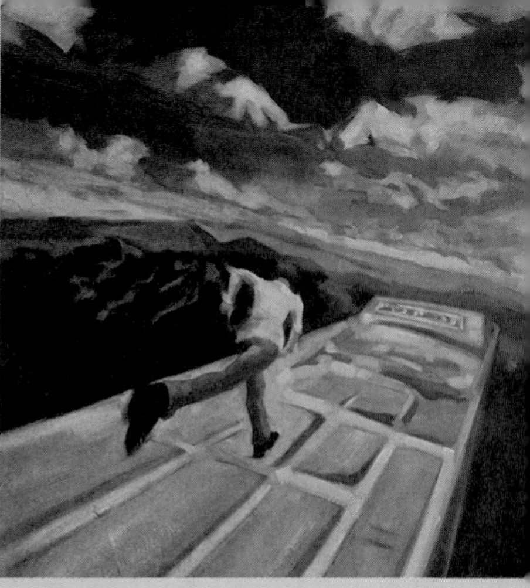

The Pharmacy Technician Series

PHARMACY CALCULATIONS

Series Author
Mike Johnston, CPhT

Contributing Authors
Jennifer Fix, RPh, MBA
Robin Luke, CPhT

The Pharmacy Technician Series
The Pharmacy Technician Series
The Pharmacy Technician Series
The Pharmacy Technician Series
The Pharmacy Technician Series

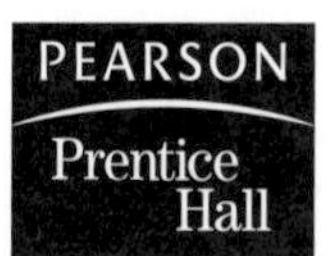

Upper Saddle River, New Jersey 07458

Library of Congress Cataloging-in-Publication Data

The pharmacy technician series. Pharmacy calculations / [edited by] Mike Johnston.
p. ; cm.
Includes bibliographical references and index.
ISBN 0-13-114740-4
1. Pharmaceutical arithmetic. 2. Pharmacy technicians. I. Johnston, Mike, CPhT.
[DNLM: 1. Mathematics—Problems and Exercises. 2. Weights and Measures—Problems and Exercises.
3. Dosage Forms—Problems and Exercises. 4. Drug Compounding—Problems and Exercises.
QV 18.2 P53687 2006]
RS57.P485 2006
615.14'01513—dc22 2005045930

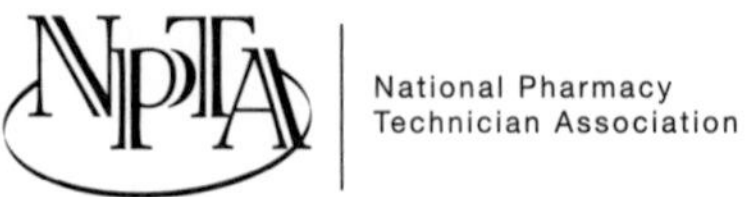

The NPTA logo is a trademark of the National Pharmacy Technician Association

straden-schaden, inc.®

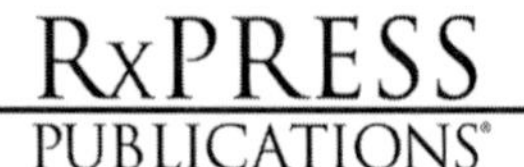

The Straden-Schaden and RxPress logos are both trademarks of Straden-Schaden, Inc.

Publisher: Julie Levin Alexander
Assistant to Publisher: Regina Bruno
Acquisitions Editor: Joan Gill
Developmental Editor: Triple SSS Press Media Development, Inc.
Editorial Assistant: Bronwen Glowacki
Director of Marketing: Karen Allman
Marketing Coordinator: Michael Sirinides
Channel Marketing Manager: Rachele Strober
Director of Production and Manufacturing: Bruce Johnson
Managing Production Editor: Patrick Walsh
Production Liaison: Christina Zingone
Production Editor: Caterina Melara/Prepare, Inc.
Manufacturing Manager: Ilene Sanford
Manufacturing Buyer: Pat Brown
Design Director: Cheryl Asherman
Interior Designer: Amy Rosen
Cover Designer: Mary Siener
Cover Illustrator: Edward Sherman
Compositor: Prepare, Inc.
Printer/Binder: Courier/Westford
Cover Printer: Phoenix Color Corp.
Photo Acknowledgment: We wish to thank the National Pharmacy Technician Association and Multi Med Media for providing the photos for this volume.

Cover Illustration: © 2006 by Edward Sherman

Notice: The author and the publisher of this volume have taken care to make certain that the doses of drugs and schedules of treatment are correct and compatible with the standards generally accepted at the time of publication. Nevertheless, as new information becomes available, changes in treatment and in the use of drugs become necessary. The reader is advised to carefully consult the instruction and information material included in the package insert of each drug or therapeutic agent before administration. This advise is especially important when using, administering, or recommending new and infrequently used drugs. The author and publisher disclaim all responsibility for any liability, loss, injury, or damage incurred as a consequence, directly or indirectly, of the use and application of any of the contents of this volume. It is the responsibility of the reader to familiarize himself or herself with the policies and procedures set by the federal, state, and local agencies as well as the institution or agency where the reader may be employed. It is the reader's responsibility to stay informed of any new changes or recommendations made by any federal, state, and local agency as well as by his or her employing institution or agency.

Pearson Education Ltd.
Pearson Education Singapore Pte. Ltd.
Pearson Education Canada, Ltd.
Pearson Education—Japan
Pearson Education Australia Pty. Limited
Pearson Education North Asia Ltd.
Pearson Educación de Mexico, S.A. de C.V.
Pearson Education Malaysia Pte. Ltd.

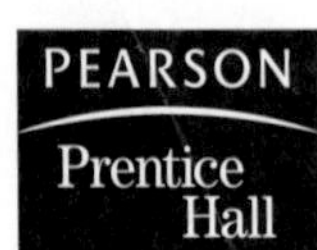

10 9 8 7 6 5 4 3 2 1
ISBN 0-13-114740-4

Dedication

To my sister . . . *regardless of the past, present, or future, I am comforted by knowing that you will continue to stand by my side, as I will yours.*

"Like branches on a tree we grow in different directions yet our roots remain as one. Each of our lives will always be a special part of the other."—Anonymous

To my niece . . . *you have amazed me since I watched you take your first breath; you've renewed my childlike spirit and continue to provide me with inspiration. Remember that life is not easy . . . it is not always fair, but I will always be there to support you—in all that you do.*

Contents

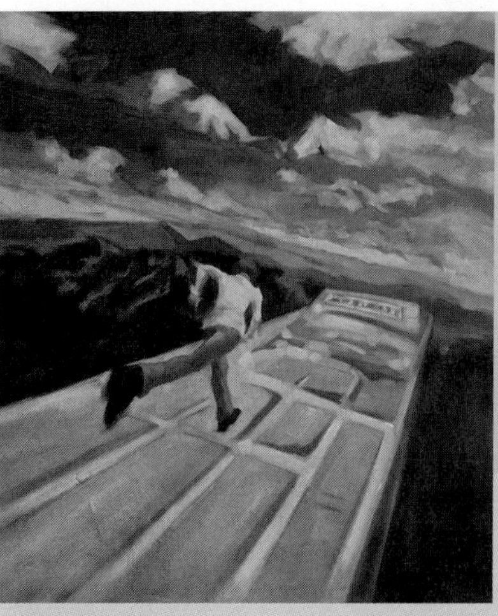

The Pharmacy Technician Series

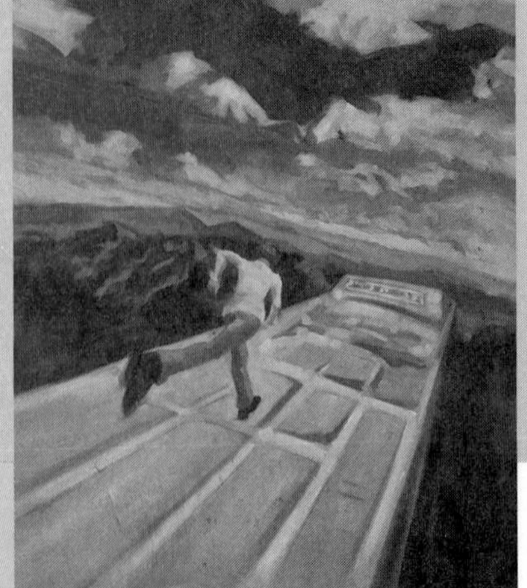

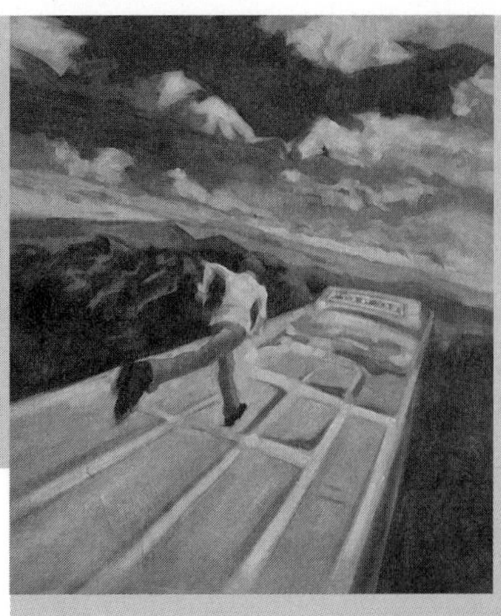

The Pharmacy Technician Series
The Pharmacy Technician Series
The Pharmacy Technician Series
The Pharmacy Technician Series
The Pharmacy Technician Series

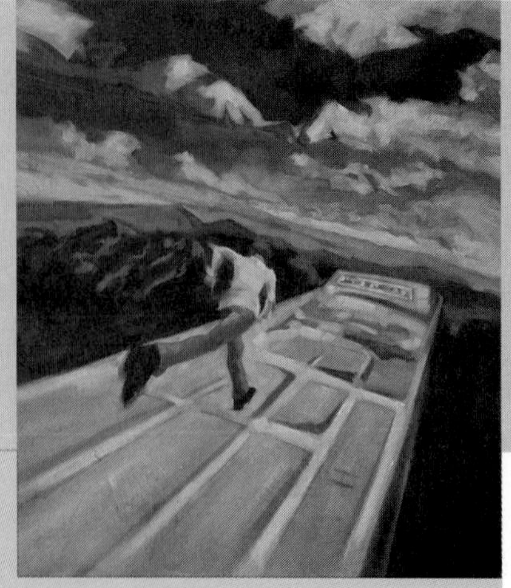

The Pharmacy Technician Series

The Pharmacy Technician Series
The Pharmacy Technician Series
The Pharmacy Technician Series

Preface

Pharmacy Calculations is a core title in Prentice Hall's newest series for pharmacy technician education. *The Pharmacy Technician Series* comprises six books that have been developed and designed together, ensuring greater success for the pharmacy technician student.

About the Book

Calculations are undoubtedly the most challenging component of training for the majority of pharmacy technician students. This book, however, has been designed to guide the student through with ease, as each theory builds on those presented in earlier chapters.

The core features of this book include the following:

- Chapter introductions and summaries provide the student with a clearer understanding and rationale of the content being covered.
- Logical, step-by-step instructions are illustrated with the use of example problems.
- Each topical subcategory provides a variety of practice problems before advancing to the next concept. This provides students with the opportunity to master their calculative skills, either at home or in class. Answers are provided to each practice problem for self-review.
- Formulas are highlighted and focused throughout appropriate chapters, allowing students to easily reference them as needed.
- Chapter reviews provide additional calculations for the student to perform and an opportunity for instructors to assess student comprehension.
- A basic math pretest enables both students and instructors to determine their initial strengths and weaknesses in theories necessary for pharmacy calculations.

- Practical examples are provided at the end of the text and serve as a comprehensive overview and learning assessment of the entire text; these are presented in problems common to actual practice settings to better prepare the pharmacy technician student.

Ensuring Content Accuracy

Numerous errors would typically be expected in a first-edition math text. Our team, however, took a unique approach to ensure the highest degree of accuracy possible. First, the majority of the text was written by a single, primary author, which provides a consistency of style, instruction, and principles throughout the entire text. In addition, during the review process, five industry experts from across the United States worked each example, problem, and question—by hand—to ensure the accuracy of selected answers.

About the Series

While a variety of textbooks and training manuals have been available for pharmacy technician education, none met the true educational needs of the industry—until now.

We set out to develop the most comprehensive, accurate, and current texts ever published for pharmacy technicians. One method we used to achieve this goal was involving pharmacy technician educators and trainers from across the country in every phase of the project. You will find that each title in this series has been developed, written, and reviewed exclusively by practicing pharmacy technician educators and practicing pharmacy professionals—a winning approach.

About the Authors

Jennifer Fix, RPh, MBA

Jennifer is an independent community pharmacy owner in Haltom City, Texas. She has been instrumental in technician development, advocacy, and training through her voluntary participation with the Pharmacy Technician Certification Board and the Texas Board of Pharmacy.

Jennifer has developed technician training programs for her local community, P*Ceutics Institute, LearnSomething.com, and the Texas Pharmacy Association. At her pharmacy, she provides patients with immunizations, diabetes care, and specialty compounding.

Robin Luke, CPhT

Robin is a founding member of NPTA's Executive Advisory Board—the elected body of leaders for the National Pharmacy Technician Association. She has more than ten years of experience in institutional pharmacy, sterile product preparation, compounding, bulk manufacturing, and management, with a specialized knowledge of herbals and homeopathic treatments.

Robin has developed a variety of continuing-education programs with a strong emphasis on reducing medication errors; she also speaks at meetings and conferences across the United States.

with

Mike Johnston, CPhT

Mike is known internationally as a respected author and speaker in the field of pharmacy. He published his first book, *Rx for Success—A Career Enhancement Guide for Pharmacy Technicians*, in 2002.

In 1999, Mike founded NPTA in Houston, Texas, and led the association from three members to more than 20,000 in less than two years. Today, as executive director of the National Pharmacy Technician Association and publisher of *Today's Technician* magazine, he spends the majority of his time meeting with and speaking to employers, manufacturers, association leaders, and elected officials on issues related to pharmacy technicians.

About NPTA

NPTA, the National Pharmacy Technician Association, is the world's largest professional organization established specifically for pharmacy technicians. The association is dedicated to advancing the value of pharmacy technicians and the vital roles they play in pharmaceutical care. In a society of countless associations, we believe it takes much more than a mission statement to meet the professional needs and provide the needed leadership for the pharmacy technician profession—it takes action and results.

The organization is composed of pharmacy technicians practicing in a variety of practice settings, such as retail, independent, hospital, mail-order, home care, long-term care, nuclear, military, correctional facility, formal education, training, management, and sales. NPTA is a reflection of this diverse profession and provides unparalleled support and resources to members.

NPTA is the foundation of the pharmacy technician profession; we have an unprecedented past, a strong presence, and a promising future. We are dedicated to improving our profession, while remaining focused on our members.

For more information on NPTA:
Call 888-247-8700
Visit www.pharmacytechnician.org

Acknowledgments

This book, which is part of a six-title series, has been both an exhilarating and an exhausting project. To say that this series is the result of a collaborative team effort would be a gross understatement.

Mark — thank you for believing in my initial vision and concept for this series, which was anything but traditional. I will always remember the day we spent in New York City talking about cover concepts and the like at coffee shops and art galleries. More important, I am honored to have gotten to know you, Alex, and now little Sophie—and I consider each of you my friends.

Joan — you are truly gifted at what you do. I am amazed at your ability to join this project at the point you did and to guide each daunting task into a smooth and successful accomplishment. I feel that your leadership has created a better final product.

Julie — thank you for taking risks (plural) on this project, compared with standard policies and procedures. In the end, your support and belief in this project have allowed a truly innovative product to be published.

Robin — your commitment to this project, to exceeding all expectations, and to developing the best training series for pharmacy technicians available has been amazing. You are a wonderful, gifted individual—but most important, I am thankful to call you a friend.

Andrew and Jenny — thank you for supporting this project, each in your own unique ways; thank you for supporting me and the entire organization. This project tested each of us, our character, and our will, and I am honored to know you both.

Most important, I wish to thank my family. The past several years have been difficult and trying, but the strength, love, and support that you've given me have always pulled me through. ***Thank you***.

Contributors

Jenny Byard, CPhT
Assistant Title Manager
Clarian Health
Indianapolis, IN

Bobbi Steelman, CPhT
Draughons Junior College
Morgantown, KY

Reviewers

The reviewers of The Pharmacy Technician Series have provided many excellent suggestions and ideas for improving these texts. The quality of the reviews has been outstanding, and the reviews have been a major aid in the preparation of the manuscript. The assistance provided by these experts is deeply appreciated.

Lisa C. Barnes, B. Pharm., M.B.A.
ACPE Program Administrator, Adjunct Assistant Professor of Pharmacy Practice
University of Montana School of Pharmacy and Allied Health Sciences
Missoula, Montana

Kimberly Brown, CPhT
Associate Director and Instructor of Pharmacy Technology
Walters State Community College
Morristown, Tennessee

Ralph P. Casas, Pharm. D., Ph.D.
Associate Professor of Pharmacology
Cerritos Community College
Norwalk, California

Kristie Fitzgerald, BS, Pharm
Clinical Pharmacist, Department of Neonatology; Instructor
Salt Lake Community College
Salt Lake City, Utah

Madeline Jensen-Grauel, BS, Ed., M.Sc
Director, Pharmacy Technician Training Program
The University of Texas Medical Branch at Galveston
Galveston, Texas

Robert D. Kwiatkowski, BS, MA
Adjunct Instructor
PIMA Medical Institute
Colorado Springs, Colorado

Herminio Maldonado, Jr., MS, BS
Pharmacy Technician Instructor
PIMA Medical Institute
Colorado Springs, Colorado

Bradley Moore, MSN
Director of Health Science
Remington Administrative Services, Inc.
Little Rock, Arkansas

Hieu Nguyen, BS, CPhT
Pharmacy Technician Program Director
Western Career College
Sacramento, California

The Pharmacy Technician Series

PHARMACY CALCULATIONS

CHAPTER 1

Basic Math Overview

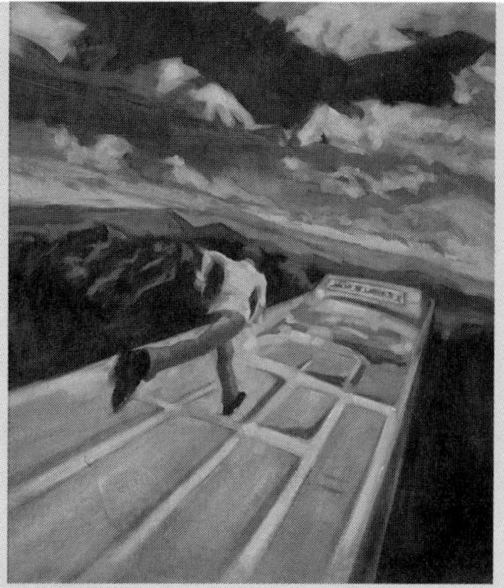

Learning Objectives

After completing this chapter, you should be able to:

- Determine the value of a decimal.
- Add and subtract decimals.
- Multiply and divide decimals.
- Change roman numerals to arabic numbers.
- Change arabic numbers to roman numerals.
- Add and subtract fractions.
- Multiply and divide fractions.
- Reduce fractions to the lowest terms.

INTRODUCTION

Knowledge of basic arithmetic is essential for today's pharmacy technician; basic skills in mathematics are required for understanding and performing drug preparations. Nearly every aspect of drug dispensing requires a consideration of numbers. All advanced pharmacy calculations, which are explained throughout the text of this book, rely on a solid understanding of basic math principles. This chapter will serve as a review of these general principles and as an assessment of your basic math skills.

Basic Math Pretest

The following diagnostic pretest will help guide your review and determine your strengths and weaknesses in basic math skills. The test should take you approximately one hour. You will need scratch paper. If you can complete the pretest with 100% accuracy, you may elect to bypass the Basic Math Overview section of this text.

DIAGNOSTIC PRETEST

Circle the decimal in each group with the highest value.

1. 4.1, 6.35, 0.31
2. 1.37, 1.33, 1.89
3. 0.4, 0.44, 0.41

Circle the decimal in each group with the lowest value.

4. 40.4, 40.0, 40.003
5. 0.15, 0.16, 0.016
6. 7.01, 7.71, 7.76

Add the following decimals.

7. 2.25 + 5.89 = ______________
8. 62.36 + 1.755 = ______________
9. 4.004 + 4.24 + 0.007 = ______________

Subtract the following decimals.

10. 8.95 − 0.015 = ______________
11. 6.665 − 0.007 = ______________
12. 18.64 − 2.11 = ______________

Multiply the following decimals.

13. 7.5 × 0.23 = ______________
14. 5.47 × 1.15 = ______________
15. 4.4 × 3.875 = ______________

Divide the following decimals.

16. 0.87 ÷ 0.2 = ______________
17. 4.4 ÷ 0.3 = ______________
18. 5.0 ÷ 5.5 = ______________
19. A jeweler had 12.5 oz. of gold in stock. Creation of a necklace required 1.8 oz. How much gold remained in stock after the necklace was made?

    ____

20. Missy Jones earned $725.78 last week. Her payroll deductions totaled $169.47. How much remained after payroll deductions?

    ____

21. Ray Wilhelm earned $371.64 for working 38 hr. How much did he earn per hour?

    ____

Identify the value of each of the following roman numerals.

22. X ________________
23. M ________________
24. L ________________

Give the equivalent arabic numbers for each of the following roman numerals.

25. XXIII ________________
26. MML ________________
27. XLVII ________________

Add the following fractions. Reduce to the lowest possible terms.

28. $\frac{2}{3} + \frac{1}{8} =$ ________________
29. $\frac{4}{9} + \frac{1}{5} =$ ________________
30. $\frac{2}{7} + \frac{1}{3} =$ ________________

Subtract the following fractions. Reduce to the lowest possible terms.

31. $\frac{1}{8} - \frac{1}{12} =$ ________________
32. $\frac{4}{4} - \frac{1}{8} =$ ________________
33. $\frac{6}{7} - \frac{1}{8} =$ ________________

Multiply the following fractions. Reduce to the lowest possible terms.

34. $\frac{1}{10} \times \frac{2}{3} =$ ________________
35. $\frac{250}{1} \times \frac{6}{9} =$ ________________
36. $\frac{5}{20} \times \frac{6}{40} =$ ________________

Divide the following fractions. Reduce to the lowest possible terms.

37. $\frac{1}{15} \div \frac{1}{10} =$ ________________
38. $\frac{2}{5} \div \frac{4}{6} =$ ________________
39. $\frac{1}{7} \div \frac{2}{3} =$ ________________

40. A jigsaw puzzle contains 5,240 pieces. Joan estimates that the puzzle is $\frac{1}{4}$ completed. How many pieces have been put in place in the puzzle?

    ____

41. There were 10,240 people attending a conference. If $\frac{3}{4}$ of the audience were women, how many women attended the conference?

    ____

42. A computer sells for $3,000. The company charges $\frac{1}{5}$ of the purchase price for a maintenance fee. How much is the maintenance fee for this computer?

    ____

Solve the following problems for x.

43. $\frac{3}{x} = \frac{5}{20}$ ________________
44. $\frac{15}{1} = \frac{30}{x}$ ________________
45. $\frac{6}{12} = \frac{x}{144}$ ________________

Convert as indicated.

46. 0.08 to a percent __________

47. $\frac{4}{5}$ to a percent __________

48. 37% to a fraction __________

49. $\frac{1}{3}$ to a ratio __________

50. $\frac{1}{500}$ to a ratio __________

Decimals

A clear understanding of decimals is critical to drug dispensing, since a decimal point can mean the difference between a correct dose and a serious overdose or underdose. To determine the value of a decimal, you must first recognize that every digit in a decimal has a place value.

Decimals are fractions with denominators of 10 or any multiple of 10, such as 100 or 1000. The value of the denominator is determined by the number of digits at the right of the decimal point. A decimal fraction is written as a whole number with a zero and a period in front of it. For example, the fraction $\frac{8}{10}$ represents the decimal 0.8, $\frac{8}{100}$ is 0.08, $\frac{8}{1000}$ is 0.008, and so on.

Remember, zeros placed before or after the decimal number do not change the value of the number. For example, 0.8 could be written as 0.8, 0.80, or 0.80000; however, in the health care profession, you should always place a zero before a decimal point to avoid misreading a number. For example, .8 should be written as 0.8 to prevent reading it as the whole number 8.

KEY POINTS

- Moving the decimal point one place to the right multiplies the number by 10. Moving the decimal point one place to the left divides the number by 10. For example, 80.65 becomes 806.5 when the decimal moves to the right ($80.65 \times 10 = 806.5$) and 8.065 when the decimal moves to the left ($80.65 \div 10 = 8.065$).
- When calculating dosages, you need to consider only three places to the right of the decimal point because drug dosages do not contain more than three digits. Figure 1-1 is a guide to place value.

millions	hundred thousands	ten thousands	thousands	hundreds	tens	ones	.	tenths	hundredths	thousandths	ten thousandths	hundred thousandths	millionths

Figure 1-1 Place Value

PRACTICE PROBLEMS 1.1

Circle the number in each group with the highest value.

1. 2.4, 3.8, 3.1
2. 4.37, 6.05, 3.34
3. 1.4, 1.63, 11.19
4. 5.4, 3.86, 10.04
5. 6.23, 7.5, 12.19

Circle the number in each group with the lowest value.

6. 0.37, 0.11, 0.19
7. 7.53, 7.54, 7.05
8. 0.1, 0.32, 0.17
9. 1.125, 0.125, 1.1
10. 5.75, 2.95, 0.06

ADDING AND SUBTRACTING DECIMALS

When adding and subtracting decimals, write the numbers vertically and line up the decimal points. Add or subtract from right to left.

EXAMPLE 1.1 Add 0.89 and 0.76.

0.89
<u>0.76</u> Add the 9 and the 6 first, then the 8, the 7, and the 1 that was carried
1.65

EXAMPLE 1.2 Subtract 0.43 from 0.67.

0.67
<u>0.43</u> Subtract the 3 from the 11, and then subtract the 4 from the 6
0.24

PRACTICE PROBLEMS 1.2

Add the following decimals.

1. 3.65 + 1.27 = ________________
2. 0.65 + 2.57 = ________________
3. 1.32 + 4.01 = ________________
4. 75.456 + 789.2 = ________________
5. 5.002 + 7.28 + 0.012 = ________________

Subtract the following decimals.

6. 402.89 − 2.9 = ______________
7. 8.1 − .056 = ______________
8. 68.22 − 4.026 = ______________
9. 2.7 − 1.0024 = ______________
10. 19.57 − 6.04 = ______________

MULTIPLYING DECIMALS

When multiplying decimals, calculate the decimals as with whole numbers. To determine the location of the decimal point, count the number of decimal places in the numbers multiplied from right to left and insert the decimal point in the answer. If the answer does not contain enough numbers for correct placement of the decimal point, add as many zeros as necessary.

EXAMPLE 1.3

$$\begin{array}{r} 0.56 \\ \times\ 0.12 \\ \hline 112 \\ 56 \\ \hline 6.72 \end{array}$$

Answer = 0.0672

PRACTICE PROBLEMS 1.3

Multiply the following decimals.

1. 5.09 × 0.5 = ______________
2. 1.75 × 3.4 = ______________
3. 4.04 × 2.25 = ______________
4. 500 × 0.015 = ______________
5. 1.3 × 4.7 = ______________

DIVIDING DECIMALS

When dividing decimals, first place the dividend (the number to be divided) inside the division bracket. Second, place the divisor (the number you are dividing by) outside the bracket. Third, change the divisor to a whole number by moving the decimal point all the way to the right. Next, move the decimal in the dividend the same number of places to the right. Then, put a decimal point in the answer directly above the decimal in the dividend. Follow the same rules as for division of whole numbers.

EXAMPLE 1.4 10.08 ÷ 2.4

$$2.4\overline{)10.08} \qquad \begin{array}{r} 4.2 \\ 24\overline{)100.8} \\ 96 \\ \hline 48 \\ 48 \\ \hline \end{array}$$

PRACTICE PROBLEMS 1.4

Divide the following decimals.

1. 0.65 ÷ 0.4 = ______________
2. 73 ÷ 13.40 = ______________
3. 0.02 ÷ 0.006 = ______________
4. 17.5 ÷ 2 = ______________
5. 176 ÷ 2.2 = ______________

Roman Numerals

Roman numerals are used in health care to designate drug quantities. Letters or symbols are used to represent numbers. The symbol and position of the numbers is the key to understanding them. Study the roman numerals and their arabic equivalents shown in Table 1-1.

TABLE 1-1 Values for Roman Numerals

Roman Numeral	Arabic Equivalent
I	1
V	5
X	10
L	50
C	100
D	500
M	1000

RULES FOR ROMAN NUMERALS

Rule 1. Roman numerals are never repeated more than three times in a row.

EXAMPLE 1.5 Five is not represented as IIIII. It is represented as V.

Rule 2. When a numeral is repeated or a smaller numeral follows a larger numeral, the values are added together.

EXAMPLE 1.6 III = 1 + 1 + 1 = 3 XXXI = 10 + 10 + 10 + 1 = 31
MDC = 1,000 + 500 + 100 = 1,600 VII = 5 + 1 + 1 = 7

Rule 3. When a smaller numeral comes before a larger numeral, the one of lesser value is subtracted.

EXAMPLE 1.7 IV = 5 − 1 = 4 XL = 50 − 10 = 40
DM = 1,000 − 500 = 500 VL = 50 − 5 = 45

Rule 4. When a numeral of a smaller value comes between two of larger values, the subtraction rule is applied *first*, then the addition rule.

Remember:

- Ones may be subtracted from fives and tens only.
- Tens may be subtracted from fifties and hundreds only.
- Hundreds may be subtracted from five hundreds and one thousands only.

EXAMPLE 1.8 The number forty-nine may not be represented by IL. It must be written as XLIX.

XIV = 10 + (5 − 1) = 14 CM = 1,000 − 100 = 900

PRACTICE PROBLEMS 1.5

Convert the following arabic numbers to roman numerals.

1. 94 ____________
2. 367 ____________
3. 28 ____________
4. 2650 ____________
5. 368 ____________

Convert the following roman numerals to arabic numbers.

6. XXXIX ____________
7. CCXIX ____________
8. DCCCXCVIII ____________
9. MCMXCIV ____________
10. XLIX ____________

Perform the indicated operations. Record the answers in arabic numbers.

11. CCXX + CD = ____________
12. MMXL − DCCIX = ____________
13. XIII × IV = ____________
14. LXVIII ÷ II = ____________
15. XIX − IV = ____________

Fractions

A *proper fraction* is a quantity that is less than a whole number. There are two types of fractions: common $\left(\frac{1}{2}, \frac{3}{4}, \text{and so on}\right)$ and decimal (0.5, 0.78, and so on). A common fraction consists of three parts: the denominator, which is the number below the fraction line; the numerator, which is the number above the fraction line; and the fraction line, which separates the numerator and the denominator. The denominator indicates the total number of parts into which the whole is divided. The numerator indicates how many parts are used or considered.

$$\begin{array}{l} \text{Numerator} \rightarrow 1 \\ \hline \text{Denominator} \rightarrow 6 \end{array}$$

FOUR BASIC TYPES OF COMMON FRACTIONS

Proper Fraction: A fraction in which the value of the numerator is smaller than the value of the denominator.

EXAMPLE 1.9 $\frac{1}{2}, \frac{5}{6}, \frac{2}{3}, \frac{9}{10}$

Improper Fraction: A fraction in which the value of the numerator is larger than the value of the denominator.

EXAMPLE 1.10 $\frac{3}{2}, \frac{9}{6}, \frac{13}{12}, \frac{7}{3}$

Simple Fraction: A proper fraction reduced to its lowest terms.

EXAMPLE 1.11 $\frac{4}{8}$ is a proper fraction that when reduced becomes $\frac{1}{2}$, which cannot be reduced further. Therefore, $\frac{1}{2}$ is a simple fraction.

Complex Fraction: A fraction in which the numerator and the denominator are both fractions.

EXAMPLE 1.12 $\frac{\frac{1}{6}}{\frac{1}{4}} = \frac{1}{6} \div \frac{1}{4} = \frac{1}{6} \times \frac{4}{1} = \frac{4}{6} = \frac{2}{3}$

BASIC RULES FOR CALCULATING WITH FRACTIONS

Rule 1. Multiplying the numerator by a positive number greater than 1 increases the value of the fraction.
Multiplying the denominator by a positive number greater than 1 decreases the value of the fraction.
Multiplying both the numerator and the denominator by the same number does not change the value of the fraction.

EXAMPLE 1.13

$$\frac{1 \times 2}{2} = 3$$ $\frac{3}{2}$ is greater than $\frac{1}{2}$

$$\frac{1}{2 \times 3} = \frac{1}{6}$$ $\frac{1}{6}$ is less than $\frac{1}{2}$

$$\frac{1 \times 3}{2 \times 3} = \frac{3}{6} = \frac{1}{2}$$ the value is unchanged

Rule 2. Dividing the numerator by a positive number greater than 1 decreases the value of the fraction.
Dividing the denominator by a positive number greater than 1 increases the value of the fraction.
Dividing both the numerator and the denominator by the same number does not change the value of the fraction.

EXAMPLE 1.14

$$\frac{2 \div 2}{12} = \frac{1}{12} \quad \tfrac{1}{12} \text{ is less than } \tfrac{2}{12}$$

$$\frac{2}{12 \div 2} = \frac{2}{6} \quad \tfrac{2}{6} \text{ is greater than } \tfrac{1}{12}$$

$$\frac{2 \div 3}{12 \div 3} \text{ or } 1 = \frac{2}{12} \quad \text{the value is unchanged}$$

REDUCING FRACTIONS TO THE LOWEST TERMS

To reduce a fraction to its lowest terms, divide both the numerator and the denominator by the largest whole number that will go evenly into them.

EXAMPLE 1.15 Reduce $\frac{4}{16}$ to lowest terms.

4 is the largest number that will divide evenly into both 4 (numerator) and 16 (denominator).

$$4 \div 4 = 1, \quad 16 \div 4 = 4$$

$$\tfrac{4}{16} = \tfrac{1}{4} \quad \text{in lowest terms}$$

CONVERTING IMPROPER FRACTIONS TO MIXED NUMBERS

To convert an improper fraction to an equivalent mixed or whole number, divide the numerator by the denominator. Any remainder is expressed as a proper fraction and reduced to lowest terms.

EXAMPLE 1.16 $\frac{23}{4} = 23 \div 4 = 5\frac{3}{4}$

ADDING AND SUBTRACTING FRACTIONS

To add or subtract fractions, change all fractions to a common denominator and then add or subtract the numerators.

EXAMPLE 1.17 $\frac{1}{8} + \frac{3}{8} + \frac{2}{8}$

1. Find the least common denominator: This step is not needed because they all already have the same denominator.
2. Add the numerators: $1 + 3 + 2 = \frac{6}{8}$
3. Reduce to lowest terms: $\frac{6}{8} = \frac{3}{4}$

EXAMPLE 1.18 $\frac{1}{3} + \frac{2}{12} + \frac{3}{6}$

1. Find the least common denominator: 12. Then convert to equivalent fractions in twelfths:

$$\tfrac{1}{3} = \tfrac{4}{12}$$
$$\tfrac{2}{12} = \tfrac{2}{12}$$
$$\tfrac{3}{6} = \tfrac{6}{12}$$

2. Add the numerators: $4 + 2 + 6 = \frac{12}{12}$
3. Reduce to lowest terms: $\frac{12}{12} = 1$

EXAMPLE 1.19 $\frac{3}{4} - \frac{2}{3}$

1. Find the least common denominator: 12. Convert to equivalent fractions in twelfths:

$$\frac{3}{4} = \frac{9}{12}$$
$$\frac{2}{3} = \frac{8}{12}$$

2. Subtract the numerators: $9 - 8 = \frac{1}{12}$
3. Reduce to lowest terms: $\frac{1}{12}$

MULTIPLYING FRACTIONS

Multiply numerators by numerators and denominators by denominators. Cancel if possible and reduce to lowest terms.

EXAMPLE 1.20 $\frac{4}{9} \times \frac{6}{8} = \frac{24}{72} = \frac{2}{6} = \frac{1}{3}$

DIVIDING FRACTIONS

To divide fractions, invert the divisor and multiply. Cancel if possible and reduce to lowest terms.

EXAMPLE 1.21 $\frac{2}{8} \div \frac{3}{7} = \frac{2}{8} \times \frac{7}{3} = \frac{14}{24} = \frac{7}{12}$

PRACTICE PROBLEMS 1.6

Add the following fractions.

1. $\frac{1}{6} + \frac{3}{4} + \frac{2}{12} =$ ________________
2. $\frac{2}{3} + \frac{1}{2} + \frac{1}{4} =$ ________________
3. $1\frac{3}{8} + 1\frac{4}{5} =$ ________________

Subtract the following fractions.

4. $\frac{5}{16} - \frac{1}{8} =$ ________________
5. $6\frac{5}{12} - 3\frac{2}{12} =$ ________________
6. $\frac{1}{2} - \frac{1}{5} =$ ________________

Multiply the following fractions.

7. $\frac{3}{8} \times \frac{5}{12} =$ ______________

8. $\frac{2}{3} \times \frac{5}{8} =$ ______________

9. $1\frac{1}{5} \times \frac{2}{3} =$ ______________

Divide the following fractions.

10. $\frac{7}{8} \div \frac{5}{6} =$ ______________

11. $\frac{1}{4} \div \frac{1}{2} =$ ______________

12. $7 \div \frac{2}{3} =$ ______________

SUMMARY

While none of the material covered in this chapter should have been considered new, sometimes you need a solid basic math overview. As you prepare to learn and understand the calculations performed in pharmacy, remember that all the calculations you will learn are based on the basic skills covered in this and the next several chapters. If you are still having any difficulty with these problems you should continue to go over this material until you have fully mastered it.

CHAPTER REVIEW QUESTIONS

Directions:

1. Carry answers to three decimal places and round to two places.
2. Express fractions in lowest terms.

Circle the decimal in each group with the highest value.

1. 4.1, 4.01, 4.001
2. 6.0, 4.5, 2.8
3. 0.2, 0.5, 0.8
4. 0.2, 0.13, 0.26
5. 3.7, 3.6, 2.35

Circle the decimal in each group with the lowest value.

6. 1.233, 1.844, 1.999
7. 4.8, 7.8, 10.8
8. 0.05, 0.5, 0.115
9. 14.03, 16.03, 12.01
10. 1.25, 3.5, 1.26

Complete the operations indicated.

11. $1.233 + 12.01 =$ ____________
12. $40.25 - 16.37 =$ ____________
13. $0.65 \times 10.467 =$ ____________
14. $31.2 \times 31.62 =$ ____________
15. $1.25 \div 0.5 =$ ____________

Convert to roman numerals.

16. 7 ____________
17. 25 ____________
18. 84 ____________
19. 67 ____________
20. 472 ____________

Convert to arabic numbers.

21. XXIV ____________
22. MMLV ____________
23. LXXXVI ____________
24. MCMXCV ____________
25. LXXVIII ____________

Complete the operations indicated.

26. $\frac{2}{4} + \frac{1}{3} =$ ____________
27. $3\frac{1}{5} + 2\frac{2}{10} =$ ____________
28. $\frac{4}{5} - \frac{1}{10} =$ ____________
29. $\frac{6}{8} - \frac{1}{4} =$ ____________
30. $\frac{5}{6} + \frac{3}{30} + \frac{3}{5} =$ ____________
31. $\frac{2}{3} \times \frac{5}{8} =$ ____________
32. $4\frac{2}{3} \times 3 =$ ____________
33. $\frac{1}{15} \times \frac{6}{30} =$ ____________
34. $4 \div \frac{3}{4} =$ ____________
35. $\frac{25}{100} \times \frac{6}{10} =$ ____________
36. $\frac{7}{8} \div \frac{5}{6} =$ ____________
37. $8 \div \frac{1}{3} =$ ____________
38. $\frac{3}{4} \div 20 =$ ____________
39. $6\frac{1}{2} + 3\frac{2}{4} =$ ____________
40. $4\frac{3}{8} \div 2\frac{2}{4} =$ ____________

Solve the following word problems.

41. A patient is to take a medication that contains 0.6 mg per tablet. He is to take 1 tablet every 2 hours until pain is relieved. If it takes 5 tablets to obtain the desired effect, the patient took how many milligrams of drug?

    ____

42. Human blood has a pH of 7.4. A urine test shows a pH of 4.6 for the urine. What is the difference in pH between the blood and the urine?

____

43. A patient takes 0.625 mg of drug twice a day for 7 days. What is the total dose?

____

44. A patient is taking 0.5 oz. of cough syrup per dose. If the bottle contains 20.5 oz., how many doses are in the bottle? ______________

45. The cornerstone of the hospital shows the date when the hospital was built as MCMLXV. When was the hospital built? ______________

46. A child is to receive X grains of aspirin. Aspirin is available in V-grain tablets. How many tablets should the child receive? ______________

47. A laboratory technician uses $\frac{1}{4}$ oz., $\frac{2}{3}$ oz., and $\frac{3}{8}$ oz. of solution to prepare an IV admixture. How much total solution does she use?

____

48. A pediatric nurse measures a 1-year-old child and finds that she is $40\frac{1}{4}$ in. tall. At birth she was $20\frac{3}{4}$ in. tall. How much did the child grow in one year? ______________

49. A pharmacy technician uses a 240-mL bottle of cough syrup to fill unit-dose vials. If each vial holds $\frac{1}{15}$ of the volume of the stock bottle of cough syrup, how many milliliters of cough syrup are in each vial? ______________

50. A pharmacist has a 12-g vial of medication. How many $\frac{1}{3}$-g doses can be obtained from this vial? ______________

CHAPTER 2

Systems of Measurement

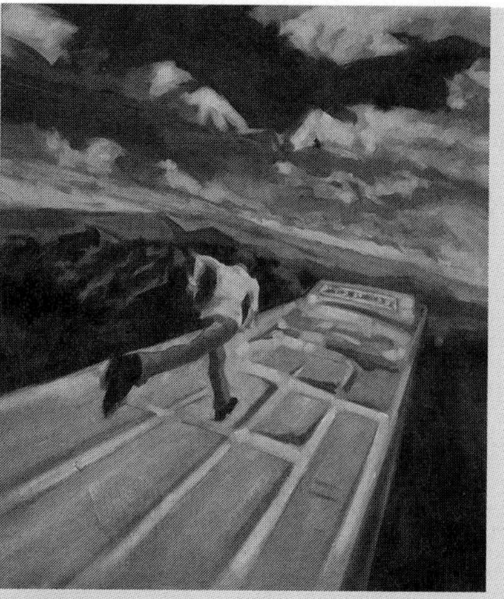

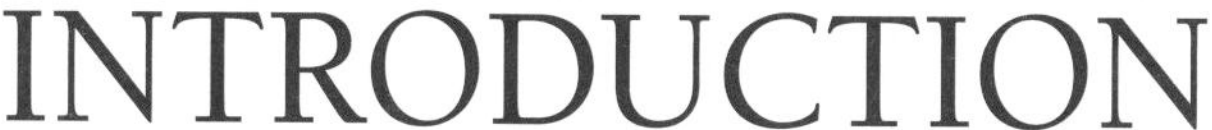

INTRODUCTION

Three fundamental systems of measurement are used to calculate dosages: the metric, apothecary, and household systems. Pharmacy technicians must understand each system and how to convert from one system to another. Most prescriptions are written using the metric system.

Learning Objectives

After completing this chapter, you should be able to:

- List the three fundamental systems of measurement.
- List the three primary units of the metric system.
- Define the various prefixes used in the metric system.
- Recognize abbreviations used in measurements.
- Explain the use of international units and milliequivalents.

The Metric System

The need for an international measurement system was recognized more than 300 years ago. In 1670, Gabriel Mouton proposed a measurement system based on the length of one minute of arc of a great circle of the earth. In 1671, Jean Picard suggested the length of a pendulum beating seconds as the unit of length. Other proposals were also made, but it was over 100 years before any decisions were made.

In 1790, the National Assembly of France asked the French Academy of Sciences to "deduce an invariable standard for all the measures and all the weights." The commission developed a system that was both simple and scientific. The unit of length was set as a portion of the earth's circumference. Measures for volume and mass were to be derived from the unit of length; therefore all units of measurement in the system were related. Larger and smaller versions of each unit were created by multiplying or dividing the basic units by 10. This feature provided a great convenience to users of the system. Similar calculations in the metric system can be performed simply by shifting the decimal point; therefore, the metric system is a *base 10* or *decimal* system.

The metric system is the most widely used system of measurement in the world today. It is more accurate than the household and apothecary systems and is preferred for health care applications. The metric system uses decimals to indicate tenths, hundredths, and thousandths. It is based on divisions or multiples of tens; thus, conversions within the system are accomplished by simply moving a decimal point.

The metric system has three primary units:

- the **meter**, which measures length;
- the **liter**, which measures volume; and
- the **gram**, which measures weight.

Prefixes are added when necessary to indicate larger or smaller units. The four prefixes most commonly used in pharmaceutical calculations are as follows:

- *kilo-* = 1000 or one thousand of the base unit
- *centi-* = 0.01 or one-hundredth of the base unit
- *milli-* = 0.001 or one-thousandth of the base unit
- *micro-* = 0.000001 or one-millionth of the base unit

Tables 2-1 and 2-2 show metric measurements and abbreviations you will encounter most frequently in everyday pharmacy practice.

TABLE 2-1 Metric Units of Measurement

Length	Weight	Volume
meter (m)	gram (g or gm)	liter (l or L)
centimeter (cm)	milligram (mg)	milliliter (ml or mL)
millimeter (mm)	microgram (mcg)	
	kilogram (kg or Kg)	

Remember: A cubic centimeter (cc) is often used to denote a milliliter.

TABLE 2-2 Metric System Prefixes with Standard Measures

	Unit	Abbreviation	Equivalents
Weight	**gram**	g or gm	1 g = 1000 mg
	milligram	mg	1 mg = 1000 mcg = 0.001 g
	microgram	mcg	1 mcg = 0.001 mg = 0.000001 g
	kilogram	kg	1 kg = 1000 g
Volume	**liter**	L or l	1 L = 1000 mL
	milliliter	mL or ml	1 mL = 1 cc = 0.001 L
	cubic centimeter	cc	1 cc = 1 mL = 0.001 L
Length	**meter**	m	1 m = 100 cm = 1000 mm
	centimeter	cm	1 cm = 0.01 m = 10 mm
	millimeter	mm	1 mm = 0.001 m = 0.1 cm

GUIDELINES FOR METRIC NOTATION

1. Always place the number before the abbreviation.

   4 mg, not mg 4

2. Place a zero to the left of the decimal when the decimal is less than 1.

   Synthroid 0.2 mg, not Synthroid .2 mg (This is a critical rule, as it will help prevent confusion and possible dosage error; in this case, 2 mg might be given if the decimal is not noticed.)

3. Never place a zero to the right of the decimal place when you have a whole number.

   A patient weighs 20 kg, not 20.0 kg

4. Always use decimals to reflect fractions when using the metric system.

   6.5 mL, not $6\frac{1}{2}$ mL

5. Avoid unnecessary zeros.

   3.2 g, not 3.20000 g

6. When converting from small units to larger units, make sure your number decreases proportionately.

   2,000 mg = 2 g

7. When converting from large units to smaller units, make sure your number increases proportionately.

   20 kg = 20,000 g

8. When multiplying metric values by multiples of 10, move the decimal point one place to the right for each zero in the multiplier.
9. When dividing metric values by multiples of 10, move the decimal point one place to the left for each zero in the divisor.
10. When in doubt, do not guess about the correct meaning. Always check when clarification is needed. A one-decimal-place error in dosing can be fatal to a patient!

PRACTICE PROBLEMS 2.1

Write the following metric measures using correct abbreviations denoting unit of measure.

1. five micrograms ________________
2. two tenths of a milligram ________________
3. sixteen grams ________________
4. five hundredths of a kilogram ________________
5. ten milliliters ________________
6. three and one tenth liters ________________
7. two tenths of a microgram ________________
8. five hundred milligrams ________________
9. six hundredths of a gram ________________
10. one hundred milliliters ________________
11. forty-one liters ________________
12. seven tenths of a microgram ________________
13. eight hundredths of a milligram ________________
14. two thousand grams ________________
15. four and one tenth milliliters ________________
16. three hundred fifty liters ________________
17. seven and four tenths grams ________________
18. one thousand micrograms ________________
19. fifteen hundred milligrams ________________
20. one and one fifth kilograms ________________

Convert the following metric units.

21. 25 mcg = ________________ mg
22. 100 mg = ________________ g
23. 0.6 g = ________________ kg
24. 1.5 kg = ________________ g
25. 0.22 g = ________________ mg
26. 1,500 mg = ________________ mcg
27. 1,000 mcg = ________________ mg
28. 15.6 L = ________________ mL
29. 1,500 mL = ________________ L
30. 0.2008 kg = ________________ mcg
31. 566.32 mL = ________________ L
32. 988 mg = ________________ g
33. 0.0125 g = ________________ mg

34. 7500 mL = _______________ L

35. 0.789 L = _______________ mL

36. 100 mcg = _______________ g

37. 6,000,000 g = _______________ kg

38. 105 L = _______________ mL

39. 2,000 g = _______________ mcg

40. 1 L = _______________ mL

PRACTICE PROBLEMS 2.2

When solving the following problems, convert everything to the same units.

1. A newborn weighs 2,800 g. What is her weight in kilograms?

   ____

2. A patient receives a prescription for 3 g of an antibiotic. The tablets on the shelf are 250 mg. How many tablets should the patient take?

   ____

3. A patient is to receive 1.5 g of cephalexin per day divided into three equal doses.

   a. If the capsules are available in 100 mg, 250 mg, and 500 mg, which dosage should be used? _______________

   b. If the dosage is increased to 2 g per day divided into four equal doses, what dosage should be used? _______________

4. A pharmacy technician must combine four partially filled bottles of powder into one. How many grams of powder does she have if the bottles contain 240 g, 0.45 kg, 2,300 mg, and 22,000 mcg?

   ____

5. How many grams of aminophylline would be required to prepare 500 capsules of 7.5 mg each? _______________

6. How many 180-mL bottles can be filled from 6.5 L of cough syrup?

   ____

7. A technician is preparing a compound. The prescription requires 350 mg of dextrose, 500 mg of sodium, and 150 mcg of potassium per 1,000 mL. What is the total weight in grams of the dry ingredients?

   ____

8. If the total dose is 0.85 g and the drug is given in four equal doses, what is the amount of each dose in milligrams? _______________

9. A wholesaler is selling 250 g of a compounding powder for $8.52. How many grams can you get for $40.00? _______________

10. You have ibuprofen tablets in 500-mg strength. If the prescription calls for 250 mg twice daily for five days, how many tablets would you give?

    ____

International Units (U)

Since a number of drugs are measured in International Units, such as insulin, heparin, and penicillin, pharmacy technicians must be able to recognize unit dosages and their official abbreviations. An International Unit measures a drug in terms of its action, not its physical weight. Do not use commas in the unit value unless it has at least five numbers—for example, 25,000 units. Remember to write out the word *unit*(s) and do not use the abbreviation IU, as it could be easily misread as a roman numeral or as an abbreviation for *intravenous*.

PRACTICE PROBLEMS 2.3

Express the following unit dosages using the correct abbreviation.

1. twenty units ______________
2. ten thousand units ______________
3. one million units ______________
4. fifty-three units ______________
5. two hundred thousand units ______________
6. twenty-three hundred units ______________
7. one hundred units ______________
8. one thousand units ______________
9. sixty units ______________
10. seven hundred units ______________

Milliequivalent (mEq)

A milliequivalent is the number of grams of a drug in 1 mL of a normal solution. Potassium chloride is a common example of a drug expressed in milliequivalents. Dosages are written with the number followed by the abbreviation—for example, 20 mEq.

PRACTICE PROBLEMS 2.4

Express the following milliequivalent dosages using the correct abbreviation.

1. fifty milliequivalents ______________
2. thirty milliequivalents ______________
3. forty milliequivalents ______________
4. five milliequivalents ______________
5. fifteen milliequivalents ______________
6. twenty milliequivalents ______________
7. eighty milliequivalents ______________
8. one hundred milliequivalents ______________
9. ten milliequivalents ______________
10. fifty-five milliequivalents ______________

The Apothecary System

The apothecary system is an old English system of measurement. Even though within a few years it will probably be replaced exclusively with the metric system, it is still used today for certain medications. The grain is the primary unit of weight in this system. The abbreviation for grain is *gr*. The basic units for volume or liquid measurement are the minim, the fluid dram, and the fluid ounce, as shown in Tables 2-3 and 2-4.

TABLE 2-3 Apothecary Weights

20 grains (gr)	=	1 scruple		
3 scruples	=	1 dram	=	60 grains
8 drams	=	1 ounce	=	480 grains
12 ounces	=	1 pound	=	5760 grains

TABLE 2-4 Apothecary Fluid Measures

60 minims	=	1 fluid dram		
8 fluid drams	=	1 fluid ounce	=	480 minims
16 fluid ounces	=	1 pint		
2 pints	=	1 quart	=	32 fluid ounces
4 quarts	=	1 gallon	=	128 fluid ounces

The Avoirdupois System

The avoirdupois system (see Table 2-5) is another system used only for measuring weight and is also being replaced by the metric system.

TABLE 2-5 Avoirdupois Weights

1 ounce (oz.)	=	4375 grains (gr)	=	28.4 g
16 oz.	=	1 pound (lb.)	=	7,000 gr

The Household System

Household units are primarily used to assist the patient with measuring while at home. Pharmacy technicians should be familiar with household measurements in order to easily explain the directions in understandable terms, such as simply telling the patient to take 1 tsp instead of 5 mL (see Tables 2-6 and 2-7).

TABLE 2-6 Household Measure Equivalents

3 teaspoons (tsp)	=	1 tablespoon (Tbsp)
2 tablespoons	=	1 fluid ounce (fl. oz.)
8 fluid ounces	=	1 cup
2 cups	=	1 pint (pt.)
2 pints	=	1 quart (qt.)
4 quarts	=	1 gallon (gal.)

TABLE 2-7 Household Measures and Metric Equivalents

1 tsp	=	5 mL
1 Tbsp	=	15 mL
1 fl. oz.	=	30 mL
1 cup	=	240 mL
2.2 lb.	=	1 kg
1 mL	=	20 drops (gtt.)

PRACTICE PROBLEMS 2.5

Express the following measurements using the correct abbreviation.

1. 50 milliequivalents ________________
2. 10 teaspoons ________________
3. fifteen ounces ________________
4. 10 tablespoons ________________
5. one hundred units ________________
6. seven drops ________________
7. two pints ________________
8. six quarts ________________
9. three gallons ________________
10. five hundred units ________________
11. ten grains ________________
12. one-half ounce ________________
13. sixteen pints ________________
14. two and one-half grains ________________
15. thirty ounces ________________

SUMMARY

Regardless of your practice setting, a solid knowledge of the systems of measurement and their units and abbreviations is the foundation for all pharmacy calculations. You must have a comprehensive understanding of this material before attempting pharmacy calculations.

CHAPTER 2

CHAPTER REVIEW QUESTIONS

MATCHING

1. centi ____________
2. milli ____________
3. micro ____________
4. kilo ____________
5. gram ____________
6. meter ____________
7. kilogram ____________
8. milligram ____________
9. milliliter ____________
10. centimeter ____________
11. microgram ____________
12. millimeter ____________
13. liter ____________
14. cubic centimeter ____________

a. one millionth of the base unit
b. one thousand of the base unit
c. one thousandth of the base unit
d. one hundredth of the base unit
e. kg
f. g
g. mg
h. cc
i. mm
j. cm
k. m
l. L
m. ml
n. mcg

TRUE OR FALSE

15. 1 mg = 0.001 g ____________
    a. true b. false
16. 1 m = 1000 cm ____________
    a. true b. false
17. 60 gr = 1 scruple ____________
    a. true b. false
18. 12 oz. = 480 gr ____________
    a. true b. false
19. 8 fluid drams = 480 minims ____________
    a. true b. false

SHORT ANSWER

20. What are the three primary units of the metric system and what do they measure?

    ________ ________ ________

21. List the three essential systems of measurement for calculating dosages.

    ________ ________ ________

22. List three drugs that are measured in International Units.

    ________ ________ ________

23. What is a milliequivalent, or mEq?

    ____

24. List four guidelines for metric notation.

    ____

    ____

    ____

    ____

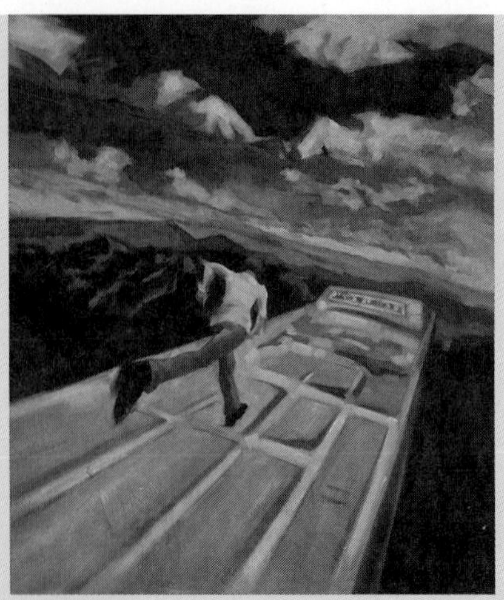

CHAPTER 3

Conversions of Measurement

Learning Objectives

After completing this chapter, you should be able to:

- Convert measurements between the household system and the metric system.
- Convert measurements between the apothecary system and the metric system.
- Perform temperature conversions.

INTRODUCTION

While the metric system is used almost exclusively, the other two systems of measurement are used in certain cases. As a pharmacy technician, you will need to convert units of measure from one system of measurement to another.

Conversion Equivalents

Since pharmacies stock only a fraction of the drugs and dosage forms available, it is sometimes necessary to convert an order to match the stock on hand. Several conversion factors will help you convert to the metric system from the apothecary and household values (see Tables 3-1 and 3-2). However, because these conversion factors are not absolute, the relationships are considered approximate equivalents. Therefore, you should choose the most direct route through a calculation. Remember, your job is to be sure the prescribed drug is delivered to the patient accurately calculated.

TABLE 3-1 Household Measure Equivalents

3 teaspoons	=	1 tablespoon
2 tablespoons	=	1 fluid ounce
8 fluid ounces	=	1 cup
2 cups	=	1 pint
2 pints	=	1 quart
4 quarts	=	1 gallon

TABLE 3-2 Household to Metric Conversions

Household Measure		Metric Equivalent
1 teaspoon	=	5 mL
1 tablespoon	=	15 mL
1 fluid ounce	=	30 mL
1 pint	=	480 mL
1 gallon	=	3840 mL
1 cup	=	240 mL
1 ounce	=	28.4 g
1 pound	=	454 g
1 pound	=	16 oz.

TABLE 3-3 Apothecary to Metric Conversion

Apothecary Measure		Metric Equivalent
15 minims	=	1 mL
1 fluid dram	=	4 mL
1 fluid ounce	=	30 mL
1 ounce	=	8 drams
1 dram	=	60 grains
6 fluid ounces	=	180 mL
8 fluid ounces	=	240 mL
16 fluid ounces	=	500 mL
32 fluid ounces	=	1000 mL
1 grain	=	65 mg
1 ounce	=	480 grains
15 grains	=	1 g
1 pound	=	12 oz.
2.2 pounds	=	1 kg

Converting the Household System

Converting between the systems is just a matter of memorizing the conversion factors and using them. Since the metric system is the most widely used, you should perform conversions to and from the metric system (see Table 3-3).

Be aware that there are minor differences between the various systems. One example to note is the pound. In the apothecary system 1 lb. = 12 oz., but in the household system 1 lb. = 16 oz.

If the system is not stated, assume that 16 oz. = 1 lb.

You can perform conversions between household and metric systems by setting up proportions as fractions and then multiplying the fractions to get the correct answer.

FORMULA **Conversion of Systems**

$$\text{Units that you have} \times \frac{\text{Number of units that you want}}{\text{Units that you have}}$$

EXAMPLE 3.1 Convert 5 tsp to milliliters.

$$5 \text{ tsp} \times \frac{5 \text{ mL}}{1 \text{ tsp}} = 25 \text{ mL}$$

EXAMPLE 3.2 Convert 3 Tbsp to milliliters.

$$3 \text{ Tbsp} \times \frac{15 \text{ mL}}{1 \text{ Tbsp}} = 45 \text{ mL}$$

EXAMPLE 3.3 Convert 4 oz. to milliliters.

$$4 \text{ oz.} \times \frac{30 \text{ mL}}{1 \text{ oz.}} = 120 \text{ mL}$$

EXAMPLE 3.4 Convert 6.5 cups to milliliters.

$$6.5 \text{ cups} \times \frac{240 \text{ mL}}{1 \text{ cup}} = 1560 \text{ mL}$$

EXAMPLE 3.5 Convert 60 mL to teaspoons.

$$60 \text{ mL} \times \frac{1 \text{ tsp}}{5 \text{ mL}} = 12 \text{ tsp}$$

PRACTICE PROBLEMS 3.1

Convert the following measurements.

1. 3 tsp = ________________ mL
2. 4 pints = ________________ mL
3. 1 Tbsp = ________________ mL
4. 3 fl. oz. = ________________ mL
5. 3 gal. = ________________ mL
6. 8 mL = ________________ tsp

7. 7 pt. = ________________ mL
8. 5 lb. = ________________ g
9. 2365 mL = ________________ pt.
10. 90 Tbsp = ________________ mL
11. 4.5 gal. = ________________ pt.
12. 45 mL = ________________ fl. oz.
13. 60 kg = ________________ lb.
14. 20 mL = ________________ tsp
15. 6 oz. = ________________ mL
16. 3 qt. = ________________ pt.
17. 5 cups = ________________ oz.
18. 1.5 gal. = ________________ qt.
19. 12 oz. = ________________ cups
20. 2 cups = ________________ tsp
21. You need to give 4 mg of a drug. The drug on hand has a concentration of 15 mg per ounce. How many teaspoons will you give?

    ____

22. The prescription calls for a dosage of 2 teaspoons. Your stock bottle contains 16 oz. How many teaspoons are in this bottle?

    ____

23. You are to reconstitute a particular drug. Each vial will get 6 oz. of sterile water. You have 2 gal. of sterile water. How many vials can you prepare? ________________
24. You need to prepare three prescriptions containing the following volumes: 1 gal., 2 qt., and 10 oz. How many tablespoons were dispensed in the three prescriptions? ________________
25. How many teaspoons are in a pint? ________________

Converting the Apothecary System

The apothecary system is an ancient system of measurement based on grains of wheat, and it allows for more approximate than exact values. Some prescribers still order medications using the apothecary system. The most commonly used apothecary measures are grains for solids and drams for liquids. The majority of apothecary-unit applications are with older drugs such as codeine, phenobarbital, and aspirin.

EXAMPLE 3.6 Convert 180 gr to ounces.

Using the conversion value, set up a proportion to solve for the number of ounces:

$$1 \text{ oz.} = 480 \text{ gr}$$

$$\frac{1 \text{ oz.}}{480 \text{ gr}} = \frac{x \text{ oz.}}{180 \text{ gr}}$$

Then cross-multiply and solve for x.

$$480x = 180$$
$$x = \frac{180}{480}$$
$$= 0.375$$

So 180 gr = 0.375 oz.

PRACTICE PROBLEMS 3.2

Convert the following measurements.

1. 5 gr = ________________ mg
2. 20 mL = ________________ drams
3. 15 gr = ________________ mg
4. 4 oz. = ________________ g
5. 600 mg = ________________ gr
6. $\frac{1}{2}$ oz. = ________________ mL
7. 7 drams = ________________ oz.
8. 9 kg = ________________ lb.
9. $\frac{1}{6}$ gr = ________________ mg
10. 40 mL = ________________ drams
11. 240 mL = ________________ oz.
12. 50 gr = ________________ mg
13. 3.5 kg = ________________ lb.
14. 60 drams = ________________ oz.
15. 150 lb. = ________________ oz.
16. 680 g = ________________ lb.
17. 99 lb. = ________________ kg
18. 0.5 gr = ________________ mg
19. 300 mg = ________________ gr
20. 1 dram = ________________ mL
21. A child weighs 45 lb. and is to receive 2 mg/kg/day. How much of the drug should the child receive per day? ________________
22. A medication order calls for a potassium supplement to be administered in at least 150 mL of juice. How many ounces of juice should the patient pour? ________________
23. A baby weighs 16 lb. What is the baby's weight in kilograms?

    ____
24. A doctor orders codeine $\frac{1}{5}$ gr. How many milligrams is this dose equivalent to? ________________
25. A cancer patient is given $\frac{1}{4}$ gr of morphine sulfate every 2 hr. How many milligrams of morphine does he receive in 8 hr? ________________

26. A pharmacy technician is to fill a prescription for aminophylline 10 gr. Tablets are available in 500 mg. How many tablets should the technician give? ________________

27. A bottle of medication contains 45 drams. How many milliliters does it contain? ________________

28. A prescription calls for the patient to take 6 drams. How many ounces would that be? ________________

29. Twenty-three grains equals how many grams? ________________

30. How many milliliters of cough medicine are in 12 drams?
____

Temperature Conversions

Another important conversion in health care involves Celsius and Fahrenheit temperature. The temperature measurement most commonly used in the United States is the Fahrenheit (°F) scale. In most other countries, the metric measurement of Celsius (°C) or Centigrade is used. In the Fahrenheit system, the freezing point is 32° and the boiling point is 212°. In the Celsius system, the freezing point is 0° and the boiling point is 100°. Simple formulas are used for converting between the two temperature scales. There is a 180° difference between the boiling and the freezing points on the Fahrenheit thermometer, and a 100° difference between the boiling and freezing points on the Celsius thermometer. Therefore, each Celsius degree is $\frac{180}{100}$ or 1.8 the size of a Fahrenheit degree. To convert from Fahrenheit temperature to Celsius, use the following formula:

FORMULA **Temperature Conversion—Fahrenheit to Celsius**

$$°C = \frac{°F - 32}{1.8}$$

EXAMPLE 3.7 Convert 80°F to °C.

$$°C = \frac{80 - 32}{1.8}$$

$$= \frac{48}{1.8}$$

$$= 26.7°$$

To convert Celsius temperature to Fahrenheit, multiply by 1.8 and add 32.

FORMULA **Temperature Conversion—Celsius to Fahrenheit**

$$°F = 1.8 \times °C + 32$$

EXAMPLE 3.8 Convert 60°C to °F.

$$
\begin{aligned}
°F &= 1.8 \times 60 + 32 \\
&= 108 + 32 \\
&= 140°
\end{aligned}
$$

PRACTICE PROBLEMS 3.3

Convert the following temperatures. Round your answers to tenths.

1. 59° F = ________________ C
2. 99° F = ________________ C
3. 100 F° = ________________ C
4. 80° F = ________________ C
5. 130° F = ________________ C
6. 4° C = ________________ F
7. 32° C = ________________ F
8. 19° C = ________________ F
9. 38.4° C = ________________ F
10. 10° C = ________________ F
11. The normal temperature of hot water is 115° F. What is the temperature in Celsius? ________________
12. The normal range for body temperature is 96.8° to 100° F. What is the range in Celsius? ________________
13. The normal oral temperature is 37° C. What is the temperature in Fahrenheit? ________________
14. If a child has a fever of 100° F, what is his temperature in Celsius?

    ____
15. If a drug is to be kept at 56° F, what is the temperature in Celsius?

    ____

SUMMARY

Every practice setting is individual and unique; the conversions that you need to calculate on a regular basis at your practice setting will become second nature to you. Until such time, use the charts and formulas from this chapter. While miscalculating a conversion may seem to be a minor issue, it could have irrevocable effects on a patient's health.

CHAPTER 3

CHAPTER REVIEW QUESTIONS

MULTIPLE CHOICE

1. 800 g = ______________
   a. 1.8 lb.   c. 8 lb.
   b. 18 lb.   d. 0.8 lb.
2. 2 cups = ______________
   a. 120 mL   c. 480 mL
   b. 240 mL   d. 160 mL
3. 160 oz. = ______________
   a. 1 pt.   c. 2 pt.
   b. 10 pt.   d. 20 pt.
4. 2.5 cups = ______________
   a. 2.0 oz.   c. 3.0 oz.
   b. 20 oz.   d. 30 oz.
5. 2° F = ______________
   a. 32.4° C   c. −12.4° C
   b. 28.6° C   d. −16.7° C
6. How many 8-oz. bottles can be filled from 5 gal. of medicine? ______________
   a. 80   c. 30
   b. 20   d. 110
7. A child weighs 45.9 kg. What is his weight in pounds? ______________
   a. 128 lb.   c. 74 lb.
   b. 87 lb.   d. 101 lb.
8. A medication has 300 mg in 50 mL. How many milligrams are in 3 oz.? ______________
   a. 900 mg   c. 540 mg
   b. 1500 mg   d. 450 mg
9. If there are 30 mg in a teaspoon, how many grams are in a fluid ounce? ______________
   a. 6.0 g   c. 0.18 g
   b. 1.5 g   d. 0.15 g
10. If a prescription reads "Take 3 tablespoons 4 times a day for 10 days," how many total tablespoons will the patient take?

    ____

    a. 240 Tbsp   c. 80 Tbsp
    b. 120 Tbsp   d. 60 Tbsp

TRUE OR FALSE

11. 110° C = 230° F ______________
    a. true   b. false
12. 12 oz. = 84 drams ______________
    a. true   b. false
13. 5 gr = 425 mg ______________
    a. true   b. false
14. If a patient weighs 204 lb., he weighs 83 kg.

    ____

    a. true   b. false
15. There are 16 2-Tbsp doses in 1 pt. of medication. ______________
    a. true   b. false

SHORT ANSWER

16. What is the formula for the conversion of systems? ______________
17. Describe a minor difference to keep in mind when converting between systems.

    ____
18. How many milligrams of amoxicillin (150 mg/5 mL) are in 35 mL?

    ____
19. If a physician prescribes 2 Tbsp. twice a day, how many days will an 8-oz. bottle last?

    ____
20. There are 65 mg in a tablespoon of medication; how many milligrams are in 8 oz.?

    ____

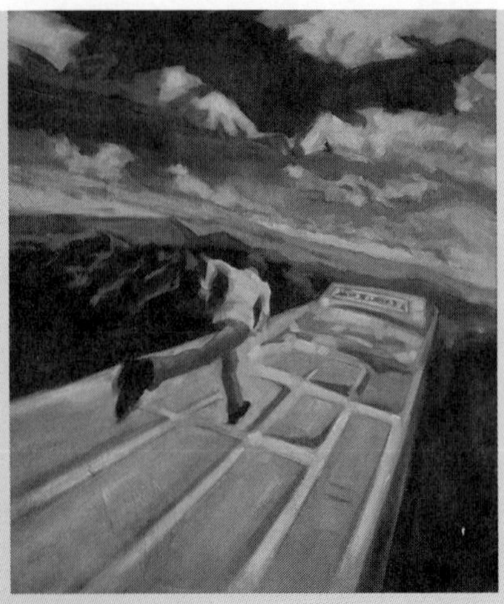

CHAPTER 4

Ratios and Proportions

Learning Objectives

After completing this chapter, you should be able to:

- Set up ratios and proportions.
- Solve ratios and proportions using cross-multiplication.
- Restate a ratio as a fraction.
- Restate a fraction as a ratio.
- Convert a ratio to a percentage.

INTRODUCTION

Technicians commonly use ratios and proportions in solving pharmaceutical calculations. Once you understand how to set up ratios and proportions, keeping units consistent, you will be able to solve most problems. Once you have set up a ratio or proportion, keeping like units consistent, then cross-multiply to solve for the unknown (x).

Setting Up a Ratio or Proportion

When solving calculations that relate to pharmaceutical products, assess the information provided and write out the first fraction using the "given," which usually indicates the strength or dosage of the product noted on the label of the stock bottle. This is usually the dose in milligrams over the volume needed to represent one dose. For example, if you have a product that is 5 mg/mL, this means that there are 5 mg of active ingredient in each milliliter. This is the same as 5 mg/1 mL.

The first fraction is followed by the double colon symbol (::).

The second fraction contains the unknown, represented by *x*, and the other element that is provided in the problem. To find out how many milligrams are in 15 mL, we can set up the following ratio and proportion.

$$\frac{5\text{ mg}}{1\text{ mL}} :: \frac{x\text{ mg}}{15\text{ mL}}$$

A key to setting up ratios and proportions is to keep like units consistent. This means that if the first fraction is stated as mg/mL, then the second fraction should be stated the same way, in mg/mL. This enables you to solve the equation and identify the answer using the correct units. Be aware of what units are needed for the final answer, such as milligrams, grams, milliliters, liters, percent strength, or rate of flow.

Sometimes the given is presented as a percent strength of a product that will need to be restated as a fraction. A percent strength restated as a fraction is always represented as g/100. For example, a 5% solution could be restated as a fraction of 5 g/100 mL. This means that there are 5 g of active ingredient for each 100 mL of solution. Likewise, a 5% ointment has 5 g of active ingredient for each 100 g of ointment. This is an important rule to remember and use when appropriate to set up a ratio or proportion.

Cross-Multiplication

Cross-multiplication is an important function to understand. Once you have set up two fractions in relationship to each other as a ratio or proportion, as noted by the double colon in the middle (::), you can cross-multiply to solve for the unknown (*x*).

EXAMPLE 4.1

$$\frac{12.5\text{ mg}}{5\text{ mL}} :: \frac{x\text{ mg}}{75\text{ mL}}$$

The two fractions set in relation to each other are $\frac{12.5}{5}$ and $\frac{x}{75}$.

To cross-multiply, identify the diagonal that does not contain *x*, and multiply those two numbers (12.5 × 75). Next, identify the diagonal that contains *x* and divide by the number shown on that diagonal (5).

$$(12.5 \times 75) \div 5 = 187.5\text{ mg}$$

Restating a Ratio as a Fraction

A ratio expresses the relationship of two numbers and is separated by a colon (:). 1 : 2 is stated as "1 to 2." This ratio can be rewritten as a fraction, $\frac{1}{2}$, stated as "1 over 2."

PRACTICE PROBLEMS 4.1

Convert the following ratios to fractions and reduce to the lowest terms.

1. 2 : 4 ________________
2. 6 : 8 ________________
3. 1 : 25 ________________
4. 1 : 400 ________________

Restating a Fraction as a Ratio

Rewrite the numerator as the first number followed by a colon (:) followed by the denominator as the second number in the ratio. The fraction $\frac{5}{8}$, stated as 5 over 8, can be restated as 5 : 8, or 5 to 8.

PRACTICE PROBLEMS 4.2

Convert the following fractions to ratios.

1. $\frac{4}{5}$ ________________
2. $\frac{9}{10}$ ________________
3. $\frac{1}{400}$ ________________
4. $\frac{1}{20}$ ________________

Converting a Ratio to a Percentage

To convert a ratio to a percentage, rewrite the ratio as a fraction and multiply by 100.

EXAMPLE 4.2

$$1:4 = \frac{1}{4}$$

$$\frac{1}{4} \times 100 = 25\%$$

When relating the percent strength to a pharmaceutical product, this means that for each 100 mL of volume or grams of solid, there are 25 g of active ingredient. If a problem states a product in a ratio strength, it is necessary to convert the ratio strength to a percent strength before setting up the equation.

PRACTICE PROBLEMS 4.3

Convert the following ratios to percentages.

1. 4:5 ________________
2. 9:13 ________________
3. 1:25 ________________
4. 1:200 ________________
5. 1:50 ________________
6. 1:400 ________________
7. 1:10 ________________
8. 4:16 ________________

Convert the following percent strengths to fractions that represent grams per 100 mL or 100 g.

9. 25% solution ________________
10. 1.25% ointment ________________
11. 0.05% cream ________________
12. 0.04% syrup ________________

PRACTICE PROBLEMS 4.4

Solve the following ratios and proportions by rewriting the ratios as fractions and then cross-multiplying.

1. $1:2 :: x:14$
2. $233:1 :: x:15$

SUMMARY

When setting up ratios and proportions, you must keep like units consistent. If the first fraction is listed as mg/mL, then you should also state the second fraction as mg/mL. You may often need to convert a percentage to a fraction for use in a ratio or proportion. Remember that a percentage stated as a fraction is always stated as g/100. Always convert your final answer to the required units.

CHAPTER REVIEW QUESTIONS

MULTIPLE CHOICE

1. Convert the ratio 1:6 to a fraction.

____

a. $\frac{1}{6}$　　c. $\frac{100}{60}$
b. $\frac{0.166}{100}$　　d. $\frac{6}{1}$

2. Convert the ratio 2:100 to a fraction.

____

a. 0.02　　c. $\frac{100}{2}$
b. $\frac{1}{50}$　　d. 200

3. Convert the ratio 1:8 to a percentage.

____

a. 0.125%　　c. $\frac{1}{8}$%
b. 8%　　d. 12.5%

4. Convert the fraction $\frac{2}{10}$ to a ratio.

____

a. 10:2　　c. 1:5
b. 2:100　　d. 100:2

5. How many grams of active ingredient are in 100 g of a product with a strength of 2.5%?

____

a. 25 g　　c. 250 g
b. 2.5 g　　d. 0.025 g

6. Convert the fraction $\frac{2}{100}$ to a percent.

____

a. 2%　　c. 0.04%
b. 50%　　d. 4%

7. Solve the following ratio and proportion:
150:5 :: x:30 _______________

a. 4500　　c. 900
b. 150　　d. 1

8. Solve the following ratio and proportion:
250:5 :: 125:x _______________

a. 6250　　c. 625
b. 50　　d. 2.5

9. Solve the following ratio and proportion:
0.5:1 :: 0.75:x _______________

a. 1.5　　c. 0.5
b. 0.75　　d. 0.375

10. How many grams of active ingredient are in 100 g of a 1:200 ointment? _______________

a. 0.005 g　　c. 0.5 g
b. 5 g　　d. 2 g

TRUE OR FALSE

11. When setting up ratios and proportions, you must keep like units consistent.

____

a. true　　b. false

12. A percentage restated as a fraction will always have the unit grams in the numerator over a volume of 100 in the denominator.

____

a. true　　b. false

13. When interpreting story problems, you should look for the given, which is often the dose in milligrams over the volume needed to represent one dose. _______________

a. true　　b. false

14. When cross-multiplying, first multiply the numbers on the diagonal that does not have an unknown, then divide by the number that is diagonal to the unknown. _______________

a. true　　b. false

15. After restating a ratio as a fraction, you should reduce the final answer to the lowest terms.

____

a. true   b. false

SHORT ANSWER

16. Describe the method for setting up ratios and proportions. _______________

17. Describe the steps for cross-multiplying.

____

18. Explain how to convert a percentage to a fraction and what units are used.

____

19. Explain how to convert a ratio to a percentage.

____

20. Explain how to rewrite a ratio as a fraction.

____

Calculating the Amount of Active Ingredient Required

It is often necessary to calculate the amount of active ingredient needed to prepare a compounded product. When you are given a percent strength, you can set up these types of problems using a ratio and proportion. Another method that will derive the same answer is to convert the percent strength to a decimal and multiply by the quantity.

PRACTICE PROBLEMS 5.1

Perform the following dosage calculations.

1. Dexamethasone sodium phosphate 0.05% ophthalmic ointment is commonly available in 3.5-g tubes. How many grams of active ingredient are in a 3.5-g tube? ______________

2. Promethazine with codeine syrup contains 6.25 mg promethazine and 10 mg codeine per 5 mL. How many milligrams of promethazine are in 2 tsp? ______________

3. How many milligrams of chlorhexidine gluconate 0.12% oral rinse are in a 15-mL dose? ______________

4. a. How many 1-tsp doses of Rx cephalexin 250 mg/5 mL are in 200 mL? ______________

   b. If the prescription specifies 1 tsp qid, how many days' supply is in 200 mL? ______________

5. Rx hydroxycobalamine 10,000 mcg/cc 30 cc Sig: 1 cc IM hs
   How many milligrams are in each dose? ______________

6. Rx estriol 75%, estradiol 25%, 2.5 mg/g 120 g Sig: Apply 0.5 g qd

   a. How much of each active ingredient is in 120 g? ______________

   b. How many milligrams of each ingredient are in each dose?

      ____

7. Rx prednisone 5 mg/0.1 g 5 g

   a. How many $\frac{1}{10}$-g doses are in 5 g? ______________

   b. How many grams of prednisone powder should you weigh to prepare the compound? ______________

8. Rx prednisone 10-mg tablets Sig: 3 tablets × 3d, 2 tablets × 3d, 1 tablet × 3d

   a. How many tablets should you dispense? ______________

   b. How many days does the given dosage regimen require?

      ____

9. Rx acetaminophen with codeine #3
   acetaminophen 300 mg/codeine 30 mg 30 tablets
   How many grains of codeine are in each tablet? ________________

10. Rx metronidazole 75 mg/5 mL
    The patient is to take 125 mg per dose. How many milliliters are necessary to provide the required dose? ________________

Pediatric Dosing

Pediatric patients, which include both infants and children, require special dosing that is adjusted for their body weight. A number of formulas have been used throughout the years to determine the best dose for pediatric patients, but the most commonly used method is stated as mg/kg of body weight.

PEDIATRIC FORMULAS

Children need lower dosages of medication compared to adults. Three formulas are used to help calculate a pediatric dosage based on whatever information is available. In some children's hospitals the pharmacy may have a preferred formula. However, the pharmacy technician should be able to calculate the correct pediatric dosage using each formula.

FORMULA **Pediatric Dosing**

Fried's Rule

$$\text{Child's dosage} = \frac{\text{Age in months}}{150} \times \text{Adult dosage}$$

Young's Rule

$$\text{Child's dosage} = \frac{\text{Age of child in years}}{\text{Age of child in years} + 12} \times \text{Adult dosage}$$

Clark's Rule

$$\text{Child's dosage} = \frac{\text{Child's weight in pounds}}{150} \times \text{Adult dosage}$$

EXAMPLE 5.3 A 1-year-old child weighs approximately 16 lb. The normal adult dosage is 800 mg. What is the child's dose using each formula?

Fried's Rule

$$x = \frac{12 \text{ months}}{150} \times 800$$

$$= 64 \text{ mg}$$

Young's Rule

$$x = \frac{1}{1 + 12} \times 800$$
$$= 61.5 \text{ mg}$$

Clark's Rule

$$x = \frac{16}{150} \times 800$$
$$= 85 \text{ mg}$$

PRACTICE PROBLEM 5.2

A 2-year-old child is running a 102° F fever. The pediatrician prescribes Tylenol and amoxicillin. The child weighs 22 lb. The adult dose for Tylenol is 650 mg qid. The adult dose for amoxicillin is 500 mg tid. What should be the correct dose of each medication using Fried's Rule, Young's Rule, and Clark's Rule?

______________________ ______________________

______________________ ______________________

______________________ ______________________

Converting Pediatric Weight

To solve pediatric dosing calculations using the mg/kg method, you must first determine the patient's weight in kilograms. To convert weight in pounds to kilograms, use the following formula:

FORMULA	Weight Conversion
	1 kg = 2.2 lb.

EXAMPLE 5.4 If a person weighs 180 lb., divide by 2.2 to find weight in kilograms.

$$\frac{180}{2.2} = 81.82 \text{ kg}$$

So 180 lb. equals 81.82 kg.

Mg/Kg/Day

When the dose is stated in the manufacturer information as mg/kg/day, this means we can calculate the patient's weight in kilograms, multiply the recommended dose, and take into account the number of times per day the dose is to be given. The goal is to determine how many milligrams can be given in each dose.

Step 1: Determine weight in kilograms.

Step 2: Multiply by the recommended dose.

Step 3: Divide by the number of doses given daily.

Using the patient from Example 5.4, an order is given for a dose stated as 20 mg/kg tid.

Step 1: The weight has been determined to be 81.82 kg.

Step 2: Multiply 81.82 by 20 mg, which equals 1634 mg.

Step 3: Divide the total number of milligrams for the day by the number of doses for the day: 1634 mg/3 = 544 mg.

Based on his weight, the patient should receive 544 mg of drug per dose.

The patient used in the preceding example weighs 180 lb. and is probably an adult. The same principles apply to calculating appropriate dosages for a child based on body weight in kilograms.

Sig Refresher

The *sig* portion of the prescription order, meaning *signa*, is where the instructions for the patient are written. Pharmacy technicians enter the information from the prescription order into the computer. The sig is an important value to remember in order to properly determine pediatric dosages. The following are some of the more common sigs you will find on prescriptions:

qd = every day

qod = every other day

da = daily

bid = twice a day

tid = three times a day

qid = four times a day

q4h = every 4 hr

q6h = every 6 hr

q8h = every 8 hr

q4–6h = every 4–6 hr

prn = as needed

Depending on the workplace, you may also see sigs such as the following:

q3d = every three days

qmwf = every Monday, Wednesday, and Friday

qw = every week

PRACTICE PROBLEMS 5.3

Perform the following pediatric dosage calculations.

1. Rx tetracycline 25 mg/kg in four equal doses

   Your patient is 10 years old and weighs 88 lb.

   a. What is the patient's weight in kilograms? ________________

   b. What is the total dosage for this prescription? ________________

   c. How much is each dose? ________________

2. Rx amoxicillin/potassium clavulanate 45 mg/kg/day q12h

   Your patient is 6 years old and weighs 68 lb.

   a. What is the patient's weight in kilograms? ________________

   b. What is the total dosage per day? ________________

   c. How much is each dose? ________________

3. Rx furosemide 1 mg/kg daily

   Your patient is 3 years old and weighs 22 lb.

   a. What is the patient's weight in kilograms? ________________

   b. What is the daily dose? ________________

4. Rx albuterol oral syrup 2 mg/5 mL 0.2 mg/kg/day in three divided doses

   Your patient is 5 years old and weighs 62 lb.

   a. What is the patient's weight in kilograms? ________________

   b. What is the total dosage per day? ________________

   c. How much is each dose? ________________

5. Rx amantadine 6.6 mg/kg/day in two doses, not to exceed 150 mg per day

   Your patient is 6 years old and weighs 54 lb.

   a. What is the patient's weight in kilograms? ________________

   b. What is the total dosage per day? ________________

   c. How much is each dose? ________________

SUMMARY

Dosage calculations are varied, and more than likely will be the pharmacy calculations you perform most often. Dosage calculations include determining the number of doses, dispensing quantities, and ingredient quantities, for both adult and pediatric patients.

CHAPTER REVIEW QUESTIONS

MULTIPLE CHOICE

1. How many 1-tsp doses are in 1 qt. of lactulose solution, USP 10 g/15 mL?
   ____
   a. 32 doses c. 128 doses
   b. 64 doses d. 192 doses
2. How many milligrams of estradiol are delivered over 72 hours by one 0.075 mg/day patch?
   ____
   a. 0.225 mg c. 8 mg
   b. 1.6 mg d. 0.075 mg
3. You are asked to compound maldroxyl 60 mL, diphenhydramine elixir 60 mL, and viscous lidocaine 2%, qs to 200 mL. How much viscous lidocaine 2% will you need to prepare the order? ______________
   a. 60 mL c. 80 mL
   b. 4 mL d. 200 mL
4. The recommended pediatric dose of ampicillin is 25 mg/kg/day q8h. Your patient is a 4-week-old infant who weighs 8.7 pounds. Which is the best dose for this patient?
   ____
   a. 15 mg c. 30 mg
   b. 25 mg d. 45 mg
5. How many days will 4 oz. of clemastine fumerate syrup 0.5 mg/5 mL last if the dose is $\frac{1}{2}$ tsp daily? ______________
   a. 24 days c. 30 days
   b. 48 days d. 60 days
6. How many grams of drug are in 480 mL of docusate sodium syrup 60 mg/15 mL?
   ____
   a. 28.8 g c. 1920 g
   b. 1.92 g d. 2.88 g
7. How many milligrams are in a 2-mL dose of prochlorperazine injection 5 mg/mL given IM for severe nausea and vomiting?
   ____
   a. 10 mg c. 2.5 mg
   b. 5 mg d. 15 mg
8. How many milliliters of chloral hydrate syrup 500 mg/5 mL are required for a dose of 100 mg? ______________
   a. 2.5 mL c. 2 mL
   b. 5 mL d. 1 mL
9. The recommended pediatric dose for promethazine is 0.25 mg/kg qid. What is the best dose for a 12-year-old male who weighs 95 lb? ______________
   a. 2.5 mg c. 12.5 mg
   b. 10 mg d. 15 mg
10. How many total grams of active ingredient are in five syringes of testosterone 4 g/100 g topical gel containing 3 g of gel each? What is the percent strength of the final product? ______________
    a. 15 g, 0.4% c. 2.4 g, 40%
    b. 0.6 g, 4% d. 60 g, 0.04%

TRUE OR FALSE

11. When solving dosage calculations, it is helpful to look for the given. ______________
    a. true b. false
12. When setting up ratios and proportions to solve dosage calculations, it is best to keep like units consistent. ______________
    a. true b. false
13. The unknown, *x*, will always be located in the upper left corner when setting up dosage calculations. ______________
    a. true b. false

14. When choosing the answer in a multiple-choice question, you should find the numerical answer regardless of units. ________________

    a. true b. false

15. You can solve most dosage calculations by cross-multiplying. ________________

    a. true b. false

SHORT ANSWER

16. Describe why proper dosing of medications is important to ensure patient safety.

    ____

17. Name three types of dosage forms.

    ____________ ____________ ____________

18. Which dose is larger, 4 mg/mL or 1 mL of 4% gel? ________________

19. How many milligrams of drug are in 0.5 mL of a cream that is 4 mg/mL? ________________

20. How many milliliters will be required to provide the necessary dose of albuterol oral syrup 2 mg/5 mL to be given 0.2 mg/kg/day tid for a patient who weighs 88 lb.? ________________

Concentrations and Dilutions

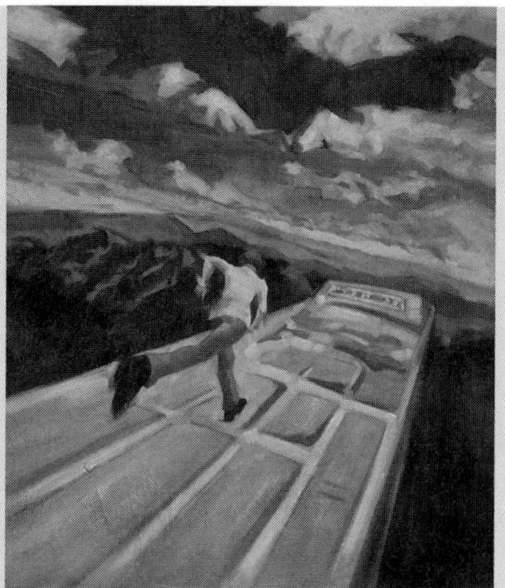

Learning Objectives

After completing this chapter, you should be able to:

- Calculate weight/weight percent concentrations.
- Calculate weight/volume percent concentrations.
- Calculate volume/volume percent concentrations.
- Calculate dilutions of stock solutions.

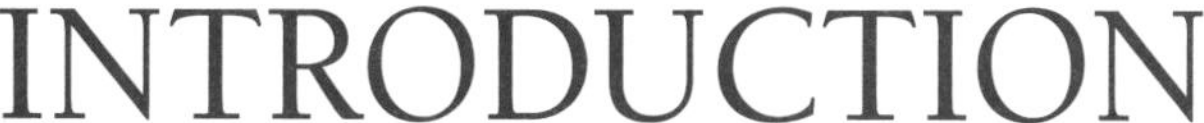

Concentrations of many pharmaceutical preparations are expressed as a percent strength. This is an important concept to understand. Percent strength represents how many grams of active ingredient are in 100 mL. In the case of solids such as ointment, percent strength would represent the number of grams contained in 100 g. Percent strength can be reduced to a fraction or to a decimal, which may be useful in solving these calculations. It is best to convert any ratio strengths to a percent. We assume that 1 g of solute displaces exactly 1 mL of liquid. Therefore, you will notice that grams and milliliters are used interchangeably depending on whether you are working with solids in grams or liquids in milliliters.

Concentrations

WEIGHT/WEIGHT

Percent concentrations for solids such as ointments or creams are expressed as % w/w. You can determine these by establishing a proportion and then converting it into a percentage, as discussed in Chapter 5.

EXAMPLE 6.1 1 g of active-ingredient powder is mixed with 99 g of white petrolatum. The % w/w calculation is as follows:

$$1\text{ g}/100\text{ g} \times 100 = 1\%\text{ w/w}$$

EXAMPLE 6.2 12 g of active ingredient is in 120 g of cream base. The % w/w calculation is as follows:

$$12\text{ g}/120\text{ g} \times 100 = 10\%\text{ w/w}$$

WEIGHT/VOLUME

Percent concentrations for liquids in which an active ingredient starting out as a powder is dissolved in a liquid, such as distilled water or normal saline, are expressed as % w/v. Again, you can determine these by establishing a proportion and then converting it into a percentage.

EXAMPLE 6.3 9 g of sodium chloride in 1000 mL of distilled water is 0.9% w/v and is commonly referred to as normal saline.

$$9\text{ g}/1000\text{ mL} \times 100 = 0.9\%\text{ w/v}$$

This is considered weight/volume because a solid is dissolved in the liquid to make a solution.

VOLUME/VOLUME

Percent concentrations that dissolve a liquid into a liquid are considered % v/v. The percentage indicates the number of milliliters of active ingredient contained in the total volume of the solution. As before, you can determine these by establishing a proportion and then converting it into a percentage, as discussed in Chapter 5.

EXAMPLE 6.4 6 mL of alcohol is diluted to make 100 mL of solution.

$$6\text{ mL}/100\text{ mL} \times 100 = 6\%\text{ v/v}$$

PRACTICE PROBLEMS 6.1

Calculate the following percent strengths.

1. 25 g of hydrocortisone powder mixed with 975 g of cream base would yield what % w/w? ________________

2. 375 mg of promethazine powder mixed with 29.63 g of PLO base would yield what % w/w? ______________

3. 25 g of dextrose in 500 mL of distilled water would yield what % w/v?

____

4. 10 mL of alcohol diluted with 90 mL of distilled water would yield what % v/v? ______________

Dilutions

Stock solutions are stronger solutions that you can later dilute to the desired strength ordered. The larger volume that you mix with the stock solution is called the diluent. You can use the following formula to calculate dilutions:

FORMULA	Dilutions
	$Q1 \times C1 = Q2 \times C2$

The equation may also be shown this way as a ratio and proportion:

$$\frac{Q1}{Q2} :: \frac{C2}{C1}$$

Notice that quantity is shown on one side and concentration is shown on the other. Note also that the initial values are diagonal to each other and the final values are on the opposite diagonal.

You should solve the equation shown in the box algebraically versus the second option of setting up a ratio and proportion. Both options will work. The secret is to place the provided elements appropriately before solving.

Where Q represents *quantity* expressed in milliliters or grams and C represents *concentration* in percent strength:

- Q1 = initial quantity (volume)
- C1 = initial concentration expressed as a percentage (stock solution)
- Q2 = final quantity (volume)
- C2 = final concentration expressed as a percentage (final solution)

Notice that Q1 and C1 on the left side of the equation represent the initial quantity and strength, and Q2 and C2 on the right side of the equation represent the final quantity and final strength. This should help you remember the equation.

In the following questions, three of the four elements will be listed; you should place them appropriately in the formula, then solve for *x*.

EXAMPLE 6.5 How much stock solution of hydrogen peroxide 12% solution will you need to make 480 mL of hydrogen peroxide 3% solution?

Q1 = x
C1 = 12%
Q2 = 480 mL
C2 = 3%

Use the formula by plugging in the known elements:

$$x \times 12 = 480 \times 3$$
$$12x = 1440$$

To solve for x, divide both sides by 12:

$$\frac{12x}{12} = \frac{1440}{12}$$
$$x = 120 \text{ mL}$$

So we will measure 120 mL of the 12% solution and add diluent qs to 480 mL. This will yield the desired quantity and strength. (*qs* means *quantity sufficient*, or as much as is needed to yield the final amount.)

Solids, such as ointments and creams, can also be diluted. If you are starting out with an active ingredient that is a powder, consider the beginning concentration to be 100%.

EXAMPLE 6.6 Rx salicylic acid 40% ointment 15 g

You have salicylic acid powder and white petrolatum. You are starting with 100% powder, which you will dilute by adding the white petrolatum.

Q1 = x
C1 = 100%
Q2 = 15 g
C2 = 40%

Use the formula by plugging in the known elements:

$$x \times 100 = 15 \times 40$$
$$100x = 600$$

Solve for x:

$$\frac{100x}{100} = \frac{600}{100}$$
$$x = 6 \text{ g}$$

So you will need 6 g of salicylic acid powder.

PRACTICE PROBLEMS 6.2

Calculate the following dilutions.

1. Rx cephazolin 2% ophthalmic drops 10 mL
   To make this order, use cephazolin injection 500 mg/10 mL vial. How many milliliters from the vial of cephazolin will be in the final preparation? ______________

(Note: Compounded ophthalmic drops must be prepared using aseptic technique in a clean room. The appropriate amount of stock solution is combined with enough sterile tear drops to make the final volume.)

2. Rx benzalkonium chloride 1:200 solution 1 L

   How many milliliters can be made from 120 mL of a 12% stock solution? ________________

3. Rx morphine sulfate 30 mg/mL oral solution 240 mL

   You have four 50-mL vials of morphine sulfate 50 mg/mL injectable. How many milliliters of product can be made using three of the stock vials? ________________

4. Rx aluminum acetate solution 1:13 dilution 480 mL

   You have a box of domeboro packets with directions stating that three packets mixed into 16 oz. of water will yield a 1:13 dilution that will contain aluminum acetate 0.48%. If the patient dilutes 1 cup of the solution by placing it in an empty gallon jug and filling with water, what ratio strength would result? ________________

5. Rx prostaglandin 20 mcg/cc 10 cc

   You have a stock solution that contains 500 mcg/mL. How much of the stock solution will you need to prepare the order? ________________

6. Rx doxepin 25 mg/5 mL 240 mL

   How much doxepin 10 mg/mL concentrate should you dilute to prepare the order? ________________

7. Rx povidone iodine 1% soaking solution 1 L

   How much povidone iodine 12% solution should you dilute to prepare the order? ________________

8. Rx lidocaine HCl 1% nasal spray 30 mL

   You have a stock solution of lidocaine HCl 4% solution. How much of the stock solution do you need to prepare the order?

   ____

9. Rx hydrochloric acid 1% solution 120 mL

   You have a stock solution of hydrochloric acid 50%. How much of the stock solution will you use to prepare the order? ________________

10. Rx hydroxycobalamine 5,000 mcg/mL 30 mL

    You have a stock solution of hydroxycobalamine 10 mg/mL. How much of the stock solution do you need to prepare the order?

    ____

11. Rx histamine phosphate 1:1000 solution 30 mL

    You have a stock solution of histamine phosphate 1:10. How much of the stock solution will you need to prepare the order?

    ____

12. Rx vancomycin 50 mg/100 mL 100 mL

    You have vials that contain 50 mg/10 mL. How many milliliters of stock solution will you need to prepare the order? ________________

PRACTICE PROBLEMS 6.3

Determine how much active ingredient is needed.

1. Rx silver nitrate 0.25% soaking solution 2 L

   How much silver nitrate do you need to prepare the order?

   ____

2. Rx thymol 4% in alcohol 30 mL

   How much active ingredient do you need to prepare the order?

   ____

3. Rx azothioprine 1% suspension 150 mL

   (Note: Once tablets are triturated to a powder, the beginning strength is 100 percent.)

   a. If the dose is 1 tsp, how many doses are in 150 mL?

   ____

   b. How many 50-mg tablets will you need to prepare the order?

   ____

4. Rx taurine 50 mg/mL 45 mL

   How much taurine powder should you weigh out to prepare the order?

   ____

SUMMARY

Concentrations and dilutions, which can appear overwhelming and intimidating, are nothing more than a series of ratios and proportions. You will use concentrations and dilutions in a variety of pharmacy practice settings, so it is important that you master this skill.

CHAPTER REVIEW QUESTIONS

MULTIPLE CHOICE

1. 50% w/w contains how many grams of active ingredient? ______________

   a. 50 g   c. 100 g
   b. 25 g   d. 5 g

2. How many milligrams of active ingredient will you need to prepare 120 mL of a product to contain 4 mg/mL of active ingredient?

   ____

   a. 120 mg   c. 480 mg
   b. 4 mg   d. 400 mg

3. What is the percent strength of clemastine fumerate syrup 0.5 mg/5 mL?

   ____

   a. 0.05%   c. 0.025%
   b. 0.01%   d. 0.5%

4. Which of the following has the highest concentration? ______________

   a. 4 mg/mL   c. 2 mg/mL
   b. 4%   d. 2%

5. What is the final volume when diluting 10 mL of a lidocaine 6% nasal spray to a lidocaine 2% nasal spray? ______________

   a. 10 mL   c. 15 mL
   b. 12 mL   d. 30 mL

6. How many milliliters of gentian violet 2% solution will you need to make 500 mL of a 0.025% solution? ______________

   a. 6.25 mL   c. 50 mL
   b. 20 mL   d. 250 mL

7. What is the final strength when diluting 25 mL of a 12% solution with 100 mL water?

   ____

   a. 5.0%   c. 2.4%
   b. 2.0%   d. 3.0%

8. What is the resulting ratio strength when you dilute 12 mL of liquid coal tar to make 240 mL of coal tar lotion? ______________

   a. 1:5   c. 1:12
   b. 1:10   d. 1:20

9. How many grams of thymol should you dilute to make 30 mL of a 4% thymol in alcohol topical nail solution? ______________

   a. 0.12 g   c. 4.0 g
   b. 1.2 g   d. 7.5 g

10. What is the final volume when diluting 100 mL of sorbitol 50% solution to a 20% solution?

    ____

    a. 120 mL   c. 250 mL
    b. 150 mL   d. 300 mL

TRUE OR FALSE

11. A solution that has a concentration of 25% contains 25 mg in 100 mL. ______________

    a. true   b. false

12. 4 mg/mL is more concentrated than 4%.

    ____

    a. true   b. false

13. One gram of solute displaces 1 mL of liquid.

    ____

    a. true   b. false

14. When using the formula $Q1 \times C1 = Q2 \times C2$, C represents concentration and should be stated as a percentage.

____

a. true b. false

15. To convert a percentage to a decimal, move the decimal point two places to the left.

____

a. true b. false

SHORT ANSWER

16. Describe the formula for calculating percent strength. _______________
17. Explain the difference between % w/w and % w/v. _______________
18. Write the formula used to calculate dilutions.

    ____
19. What is the diluent? _______________
20. What is normal saline? _______________

Alligations

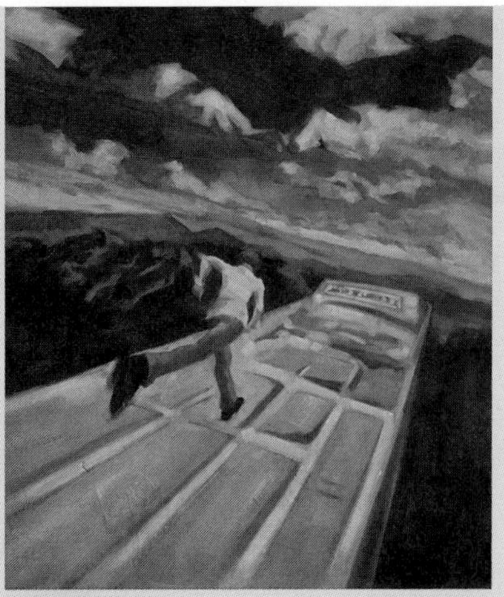

Learning Objectives

After completing this chapter, you should be able to:

- Understand when to use the alligation principle for calculations.
- Calculate a variety of alligation-related problems.

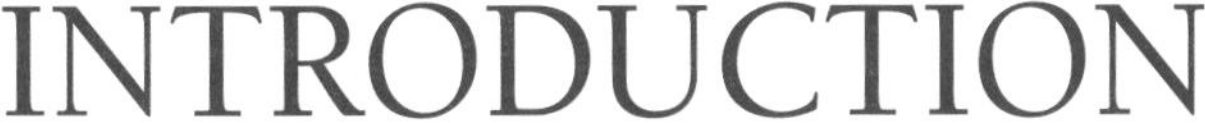

INTRODUCTION

Alligations are used when mixing two products with different percent strengths of the same active ingredient. The strength of the final product will fall between the strengths of each original product.

Solving Alligations

You can use the alligation method to determine how many parts of the same product, with different strengths, you will need to create the final strength requested. Further, you can calculate exactly how many milliliters or grams you need of each beginning product.

The Alligation Grid

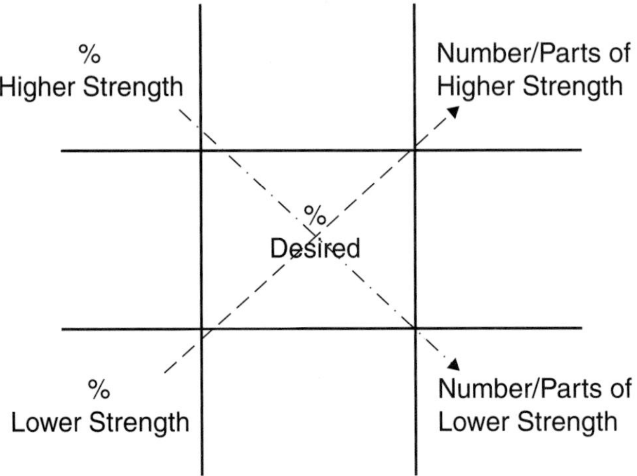

Alligation Tips

- Solvents and diluents such as water, vanishing cream base, and white petrolatum are considered a percent strength of zero.
- Liquids, including solutions, syrups, elixirs, and even lotions, are expressed in milliliters.
- Solids are expressed in grams. This would include powders, creams, and ointments.
- The alligation formula requires that you express the strength as a percentage when setting up the problem. You would have to convert a ratio strength given in the question to a percent strength.
- When writing percents or using decimals, always use a leading zero: 0.25%. This helps prevent errors in interpretation. It would be a terrible error and possibly even fatal to dispense something in 25% that was really supposed to be 0.25%.
- 1 fl. oz. = 29.57 mL. This is commonly rounded to 30 mL.
- 1 avoirdupois oz. = 28.35 g. This measurement, used for solids, is also commonly rounded to 30 g.

EXAMPLE 7.1 Rx hydrocortisone 2% ointment 120 g

You have a 1-lb. jar of hydrocortisone 1% ointment and a 1-lb. jar of hydrocortisone 2.5% ointment. The prescription is for hydrocortisone 2% ointment. Since you don't have any of the desired strength in stock, you will need to mix some of each of the strengths you have available. How many grams of each will you need to prepare the order?

When setting up an alligation, always start on the left of the page and work the problem horizontally across the page.

First, draw the alligation grid.

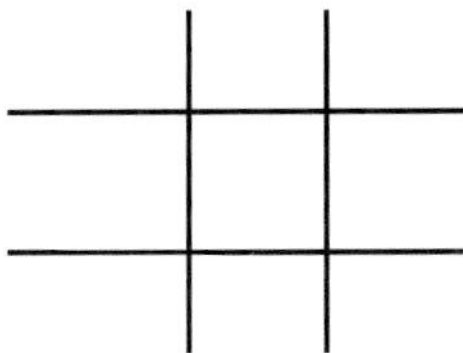

- Write in the higher beginning strength in the top left box and the lower beginning strength in the lower left box.
- Write the desired strength in the middle box.
- Take the difference on the diagonal from lower left to upper right, and write the result in the upper right box.

1 from 2 = 1 This is how many parts of the 2.5% ointment are needed (1 part)

When figuring the difference on the diagonal, always write down a positive number.

- Take the difference on the diagonal from the upper left box to the lower right box, and write the result in the lower right box.

2 from 2.5 = 0.5 This is how many parts of the 1% ointment are needed (0.5 part)

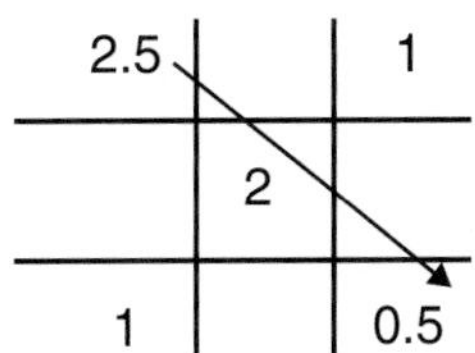

- Next, add the numbers in the third column.

1 + 0.5 = 1.5 The total of the third column is how many total parts are needed for the preparation. (1.5 total parts)

2.5 1
2
1 0.5

There will be a total of 1.5 parts.

1 part of the total will be the 2.5% ointment.

0.5 part of the total will be the 1% ointment.

- Next, write out the fractions of the total. This is how many parts of the first percent strength over the total parts. Following along the top row of numbers, representing the 2.5% ointment, write out the fraction of parts over the total parts. This is the number in the top right box over the total of the third column.

1 part/1.5 parts

- Then, for the lower row of numbers representing the 1% ointment, write out the fraction over the total. This is how many parts of the 1% ointment over the total parts. This is the number in the lower right box over the total of the third column.

0.5 part/1.5 parts

- Next, multiply each of these by the total volume you wish to prepare, which is 120 g.

Representing the 2.5% ointment the top row, calculate the following:

$$\frac{1}{5} \times 120 \text{ g} = 80 \text{ g}$$

Representing the 1% ointment in the lower row, calculate the following:

$$\frac{0.5}{1.5} \times 120 \text{ g} = 40 \text{ g}$$

This problem looks like this across the page:

$\frac{1}{1.5} \times 120$ g $= 80$ g of the 2.5% ointment is needed.

$\frac{0.5}{1.5} \times 120$ g $= 40$ g of the 1% ointment is needed.

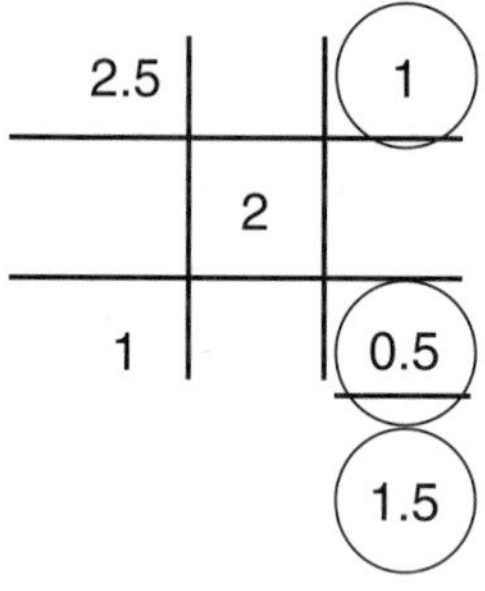

Notice that 80 + 40 = 120 g. This is a quick check. Notice also that the total needed is 120 g and if you use 80 g of the first ointment, then the amount needed of the second ointment is 120 − 80 = 40 g.

The practicality of this method is that the pharmacy can use existing stock without having to purchase additional product. The requested strength also may not be commercially available.

EXAMPLE 7.2 Rx triamcinolone 0.05% cream 90 g

You have in stock 1-lb. each of triamcinolone 0.025% cream and triamcinolone 0.1% cream. How many grams of each will you need to prepare the order?

Set up the problem left to right across the page.

$$\frac{0.025}{0.075} \times 90 \text{ g} = 30 \text{ g of the 0.1\% cream}$$

$$\frac{0.05}{0.075} \times 90 \text{ g} = 60 \text{ g of the 0.025\% cream}$$

0.1		0.025
	0.05	
0.025		0.05
		0.075

Notice that 30 + 60 = 90 g. This is a quick check. Note also that the resulting strength is between the two original strengths. The final strength of this product is 0.05%.

See how each calculation in Example 7.2 relates back to the same line. 30 g needed relates back to the top line and the 60 g needed relates back to the lower line, 0.1% and 0.025% respectively. If you work the problem across the page from left to right, then you can visually see the answer relating to the top line or the bottom line. Read across horizontally.

Looking at the calculations in Example 7.2, how many total parts are needed?

Total parts = 0.075 (total of third column)

How many parts of the 0.1% cream are needed?

0.025 (upper right box)

How many parts of the 0.025% cream are needed?

0.05 (lower right box)

What is the final strength of the product?

0.05% (center box)

How much 0.1% cream was needed?

30 g (answer on top line)

How much of the 0.025% cream was needed?

60 g (answer on lower line)

Occasionally there is a known quantity of one of the strengths and we need to find out how much of the second strength will be added to make the desired strength. The easiest way to solve this is to set up an alligation, determine the parts needed of each strength, then set up a ratio and proportion using the quantity given that relates to the appropriate strength.

EXAMPLE 7.3 How much 2.5% cream should you add to 100 g of 0.5% cream to make 1% cream?

$$\frac{1.5 \text{ parts}}{100 \text{ g}} = \frac{0.5 \text{ part}}{x \text{ g}}$$

$$x = 33.33 \text{ g}$$

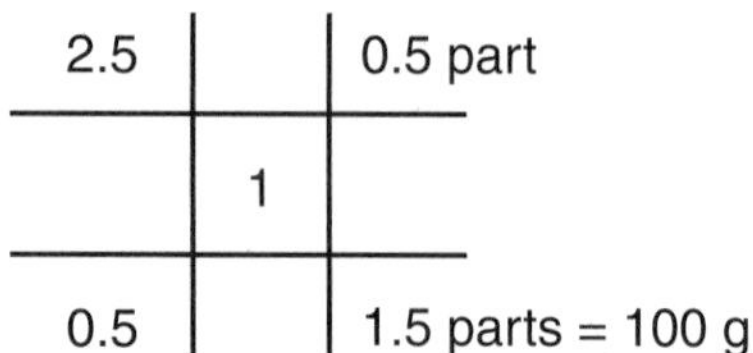

PRACTICE PROBLEMS 7.1

Calculate the following alligations.

1. Rx silver nitrate 0.25% solution 1 L

   You have a gallon of silver nitrate 1% stock solution, which you will dilute with distilled water. How many milliliters of each will you need to make the final product? Note that the percent strength of water is zero. ________________ ________________

2. Rx soaking solution 1 : 100 1 L

   You have a 1 : 25 stock solution and water. How many milliliters of each will you need to make the final product? ________________

   ____

3. Rx coal tar 5% ointment 120 g

   You have coal tar 10% ointment and coal tar 2% ointment. How many grams of each will you use to prepare the final product?

   ________________ ________________

4. Convert 1 : 75 to a percent strength. ________________
5. Convert 1 : 20 to a percent strength. ________________
6. Convert 2% to a ratio strength. ________________
7. Convert 33% to a ratio strength. ________________
8. Convert 25% to a ratio strength. ________________
9. Rx alcohol 30%

   How many milliliters of 90% alcohol should you add to 25 mL of 10% alcohol to make 30% alcohol? ________________

10. Rx hydrocortisone 2% ointment

    How many grams of petrolatum should you add to 30 g of hydrocortisone 2.5% ointment to reduce its strength to 2.0%? The percent strength of petrolatum is zero. ________________

11. Rx normal saline

    How many milliliters of water must you add to 500 mL of a 10% stock solution of sodium chloride to make a batch of normal saline (sodium chloride 0.9% solution)? ________________

12. Rx ichthammol 5% ointment

    How many grams of ichthammol 10% ointment should you add to 20 g of ichthammol 2% ointment to make ichthammol 5% ointment?

    ____

13. Rx benzalkonium chloride 1:1000 solution

    How many milliliters of water should you add to 50 mL of benzalkonium chloride 0.25% solution to prepare the order?

    ____

14. Rx zinc oxide 10% ointment 45 g

    How many grams of zinc oxide 20% ointment and zinc oxide 5% ointment should you mix to prepare the order? ________________

    ____

15. Rx aluminum acetate 1:400 solution 1 gallon

    How many milliliters of Burrow's solution (aluminum acetate 5%) should you use to prepare the order? ________________

16. Rx histamine phosphate 1:10,000 solution 10 mL

    How many milliliters of a histamine phosphate 1:10 solution do you need to prepare the order? ________________

17. Rx benzocaine 5% ointment 2 oz.

    How many grams of benzocaine 2% ointment should you mix with 22.5 g of benzocaine 10% ointment to prepare the order?

    ____

SUMMARY

In certain situations, a pharmacy must use the alligation method to combine two varying strengths of a drug or combine a drug with a base or diluent to achieve the prescribed strength. While these calculations can be confusing at first, once you master the alligation grid you should be able to perform these calculations easily.

CHAPTER 7

CHAPTER REVIEW QUESTIONS

MULTIPLE CHOICE

1. How much 20% cream should you add to 26 g of 1% cream to make a 4% cream?

____

a. 6.00 g
b. 5.20 g
c. 4.88 g
d. 3.00 g

2. How much 25% stock solution and distilled water will you need to make 1 L of a 1:400 solution? _______________

a. 10 mL of the 25% solution and 990 mL of water
b. 100 mL of the 25% solution and 900 mL of water
c. 990 mL of the 25% solution and 10 mL of water
d. 900 mL of the 25% solution and 10 mL of water

3. How much 10% cream and a 0.5% cream will you need to prepare 120 g of a 2.5% cream?

____

a. 20 g of the 10% cream and 100 g of the 0.5% cream
b. 100 g of the 10% cream and 20 g of the 0.5% cream
c. 25 g of the 10% cream and 95 g of the 0.5% cream
d. 95 g of the 10% cream and 25 g of the 0.5% cream

4. How much povidone iodine 20% solution and water will you need to make 500 mL of a povidone iodine 3% rinse? _______________

____

a. 75 mL of the 20% solution and 425 mL of water
b. 425 mL of the 20% solution and 25 mL of water
c. 20 mL of the 20% solution and 480 mL of water
d. 480 mL of the 20% solution and 20 mL of water

5. How much lidocaine 0.5% topical gel should you mix with lidocaine 10% topical gel to make 15 g of a lidocaine 2% topical gel?

____

a. 2.4 g
b. 5.0 g
c. 9.5 g
d. 12.6 g

6. How much 1:25 solution and 1:500 solution should you mix to make 1 L of a 1:250 soaking solution? _______________

a. 947 mL of the 1:25 solution and 53 mL of the 1:500 solution
b. 53 mL of the 1:25 solution and 947 mL of the 1:500 solution
c. 250 mL of the 1:25 solution and 750 of the 1:500 solution
d. 750 mL of the 1:25 solution and 250 mL of the 1:500 solution

7. Convert 50% to a ratio strength.

____

a. 1:2
b. 1:4
c. 1:6
d. 1:8

8. How much NaCl 10% stock solution should you add to 100 mL of NaCl 0.45% solution to make normal saline? _______________

a. 1 mL
b. 2 mL
c. 5 mL
d. 10 mL

9. How many grams of 0.1% cream should you mix with 12 g of 12% cream to make a 6% cream? _______________

a. 10 g
b. 12 g
c. 24 g
d. 33 g

10. How many parts of each of a 1% product and a 3% product do you need to make a 2.5% product?

_______________ _______________

   a. 2.5 parts of the 1% product and 1 part of the 3% product
   b. 1 part of the 1% product and 2.5 parts of the 3% product
   c. 1.5 parts of the 1% product and 0.5 part of the 3% product
   d. 0.5 part of the 1% product and 1.5 parts of the 3% product

TRUE OR FALSE

11. When using the alligation method, you must consider three different percent strengths: the beginning strength of each ingredient and the final strength. _______________

   a. true b. false

12. When using the alligation method, the final strength will be a value between the beginning two strengths. _______________

   a. true b. false

13. Distilled water, with a percent strength of zero, is sometimes used as a beginning ingredient in alligation problems. _______________

   a. true b. false

14. When setting up an alligation, you should convert any ratio strengths given to percent strengths before setting up the formula.

____

   a. true b. false

15. Amounts needed of powders, creams, and ointments are expressed in milligrams.

____

   a. true b. false

SHORT ANSWER

16. Describe the principle of alligations.

____

17. List three tips for performing alligations.

____

____

____

18. Describe how to verify your answer when solving alligations.

____

19. Describe how to convert a ratio strength to a percent strength.

____

20. Describe how to convert a percent strength to a ratio strength.

____

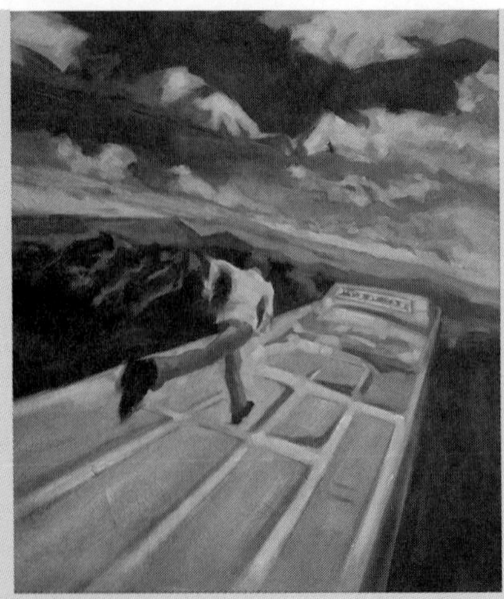

CHAPTER 8

Flow Rates

Learning Objectives

After completing this chapter, you should be able to:

- Define flow rates.
- Illustrate the dimensional analysis for flow rates.
- Calculate flow rates to determine drops/minute.
- Calculate flow rates in milliliters/hour.

INTRODUCTION

Flow rates are calculated to determine at what rate, usually stated in drops per minute, a medication will flow through IV tubing to the patient. Dimensional analysis is commonly used to perform these calculations. Dimensional analysis uses logical sequencing and placement of units so that they can be canceled out to leave the desired terms for the final answer.

Calculating Flow Rates

You could work out flow rates by using a series of ratios and proportions; however, dimensional analysis enables you to work these problems more efficiently.

When setting up the information provided in calculating flow rates, use the following formula and insert the appropriate values.

FORMULA Dimensional Analysis for Flow Rates

$$\frac{\text{Volume} \times \text{Drops} \times 1\text{ hr}}{\text{Hours} \times 1\text{ mL} \times 60\text{ min}} = \text{drops/minute}$$

ELEMENTS OF THE FORMULA

- The first segment represents milliliter/hour.
- The second segment represents drops/milliliter. This could vary depending on the IV administration set that is used. Always assume 60 gtt./1 mL unless otherwise stated.
- The third segment is always stated as 1 hr/60 min. This enables you to cancel out the necessary units so that your final answer will be solved as gtt./min.

Once the elements are placed in the formula, you can cancel out units and, if you wish, any appropriate numerical values. Multiply across the top row of numbers and multiply across the bottom row of numbers, then divide the numerator by the denominator.

EXAMPLE 8.1 Rx D5W 1 L over 6 hr

What is the flow rate in drops/minute?

Step 1: Draw the formula and place the appropriate values:

$$\frac{1000\text{ mL} \times 60\text{ gtt.} \times 1\text{ hr}}{6\text{ hr} \times 1\text{ mL} \times 60\text{ min}} = \text{gtt./min}$$

Step 2: Cancel out like units. Milliliters and hours will cancel out to leave the desired units of gtt./min.

Step 3: Multiply across the top row:

$$1000 \times 60 \times 1 = 60{,}000$$

Multiply across the bottom row:

$$6 \times 1 \times 60 = 3600$$

Divide the numerator by the denominator:

$$\frac{60{,}000}{3600} = 16.67\text{ gtt./min}$$

Since drops cannot be delivered in fractions, the answer to this question would be 17 gtt./min.

When calculating the flow rate in gtt./min, use the preceding formula. You can solve similar problems by using the information given to set up ratios and proportions. Place the given information on the left side as a fraction, followed by the double colon (::) symbol. The units on the right side must be consistent with the units on the left side. Cross-multiply to solve for the unknown, *x*.

EXAMPLE 8.2 Rx vancomycin 500 mg/250 mL 500 mg over 3 hr tid

a. How many milligrams will the patient receive per hour?
Set up the ratio and proportion.

$$\frac{500 \text{ mg}}{3 \text{ hr}} = \frac{x \text{ mg}}{1 \text{ hr}}$$

Then cross-multiply and solve for *x*:

$$x = 167 \text{ mg/hr}$$

b. How many milliliters will the patient receive in 24 hr?
Set up the ratio and proportion:

$$\frac{250 \text{ mL}}{1 \text{ dose}} = \frac{x \text{ mL}}{3 \text{ doses}}$$

Then cross-multiply and solve for *x*:

$$x = 750 \text{ mL}$$

c. What is the flow rate in mL/hr?
Reduce the proportion by dividing:

250 mL/3 hr reduces to 83.3 mL/hr

PRACTICE PROBLEMS 8.1

Solve the following flow rate problems.

1. Rx Claforan (cefotaxime) 500 mg/50 mL IV 50 mg/kg/dose
The patient weighs 22 lb.
   a. How many milligrams per dose should the patient receive?
   ____
   b. How many minutes will it take to administer the IV if the administration set is calibrated at 20 gtt./mL and the flow rate is set at 30 gtt./min? ________________
2. Rx ampicillin 0.5 g/100 mL 50 mg/kg/day q8h over 90 min
The patient weighs 30 kg.
   a. How many milligrams are needed for each dose? ________________
   b. What is the flow rate in gtt./min? ________________
   c. What is the flow rate in mL/hr? ________________
3. Rx penicillin G potassium 20,000,000 U/1 L 250,000 U/kg/day up to 20,000,000 U/day over 24 hours
The patient weighs 189 lb.
   a. What is the patient's weight in kilograms? ________________
   b. How many units will be needed daily? ________________

c. What is the flow rate in mL/hr? _______________

d. How many units will be administered per hour? _______________

4. Rx dexamethasone sodium phosphate 0.25 mg/kg/dose q8h over 15 min

   The patient weighs 14 lb. You have a stock vial containing 4 mg/mL in a 10-mL vial. The IV bag holds 50 mL and the IV administration set delivers 30 gtt./mL.

   a. What is the patient's weight in kilograms? _______________

   b. What is the dose in milligrams? _______________

   c. How many milliliters will you need from the stock vial to provide the dose? _______________

   d. What is the flow rate in gtt./min? _______________

5. Rx Ringer's solution 500 mL

   If the flow rate is set at 63 mL/hr, how many hours will it take to administer the solution? _______________

6. Rx D5W 60 mL/hr

   How many milliliters of D5W do you need for 24 hr? _______________

7. Rx electrolyte solution 500 mL

   The IV administration set delivers 20 gtt./mL and the flow rate is set at 40 gtt./min. What is the infusion time in hours? _______________

8. Rx antibiotic 250 mL over 2 hr

   The IV administration set delivers 15 gtt./mL.

   a. What is the flow rate in gtt./min? _______________

   b. What is the flow rate in mL/hr? _______________

9. Rx Rocephin (ceftriaxone) 2 g/100 mL

   The IV administration set delivers 30 gtt./mL and the flow rate is set at 60 gtt./min.

   a. What is the infusion time in hours? _______________

   b. How much drug will be delivered each minute in mg/min?

   ____

   c. Determine mg/mL. _______________

10. Rx insulin 100 U/250 mL 100 U over 2.5 hr

    The IV administration set delivers 30 gtt./mL.

    a. What is the flow rate in gtt./min? _______________

    b. How many units of insulin will be delivered per minute?

    ____

SUMMARY

Often described as one of the most challenging calculations used in pharmacy, flow rates are simply a series of basic fundamental calculations. Using ratios and proportions, which you covered earlier in the book, you should now be able to solve more complicated and in-depth calculations such as those presented in this chapter.

CHAPTER REVIEW QUESTIONS

MULTIPLE CHOICE

1. You have a stock vial of cefatazime 500 mg/10 mL. The dose is 2 g over 30 min. How many mg/min will the patient receive?

____

a. 17 mg/min c. 47 mg/min
b. 27 mg/min d. 67 mg/min

2. You have a stock vial of cefataxime 500 mg/10 mL. The dose is 2 g over 30 min. What is the flow rate in mL/hr?

____

a. 40 mL/hr c. 80 mL/hr
b. 60 mL/hr d. 100 mL/hr

3. You have a stock vial of cefataxime 500 mg/10 mL. The dose is 2 g over 30 min. What is the flow rate in gtt./min if the IV administration set is calibrated to deliver 20 gtt./mL? _______________

a. 27 gtt./min c. 80 gtt./min
b. 67 gtt./min d. 87 gtt./min

4. What is the flow rate in gtt./min for a 1-L TPN over 12 hr if the IV administration set is calibrated to deliver 30 gtt./mL?

____

a. 42 gtt./min c. 12 gtt./min
b. 30 gtt./min d. 60 gtt./min

5. What is the flow rate in gtt./min for 50 mL of an antibiotic administered over 60 min?

____

a. 30 gtt./min c. 60 gtt./min
b. 50 gtt./min d. 83 gtt./min

6. You have an order for cefuroxime 1.5 g/50 mL with a maximum dose of 1.5 g q8h. The patient weighs 200 lb. What is the flow rate in gtt./min if the dose is administered over 90 min?

____

a. 90 gtt./min c. 40 gtt./min
b. 50 gtt./min d. 33 gtt./min

7. You have a stock vial of product 30 mg/mL. How many milliliters will you need to prepare an IV containing a dose of 150 mg/50 mL?

____

a. 5 mL c. 20 mL
b. 10 mL d. 30 mL

8. The recommended dose for a drug is 20 mg/kg/day qid. The patient weighs 220 lb. What is the dose for this patient?

____

a. 0.5 g c. 2.0 g
b. 1.0 g d. 4.0 g

9. You have a stock vial of product 25 mg/mL. The dose is 250 mg. How many milliliters are required? _______________

a. 2.5 mL c. 10 mL
b. 5.0 mL d. 25 mL

10. What is the flow rate for a 250-mL IV to be administered over 2 hr? _______________

a. 125 gtt./min c. 12.5 gtt./min
b. 250 gtt./min d. 60 gtt./min

TRUE OR FALSE

11. Dimensional analysis is an efficient way to calculate flow rates. _______________

a. true b. false

12. When setting up flow rate problems, always assume that the IV administration set delivers 60 gtt./min unless otherwise stated in the problem. ______________

    a. true   b. false

13. The formula to calculate a patient's weight in kilograms is Pounds/2.2 = Kilograms.

    ____

    a. true   b. false

14. The flow rate is usually stated as mg/min.

    ____

    a. true   b. false

15. Infusion time should be stated in hours.______________

    a. true   b. false

SHORT ANSWER

16. What is dimensional analysis?

    ____

17. Write out the formula for flow rates using dimensional analysis.

    ____

18. Compare the doses needed for each of the following orders and indicate which one is the larger dose for a 10-kg patient. ______________

    Order A = 50 mg/kg/dose

    Order B = 150 mg/kg/day divided into three doses

19. A standard IV administration set is calibrated to deliver how many gtt./mL? ______________
20. Describe the first segment of the flow rate formula.

    ____

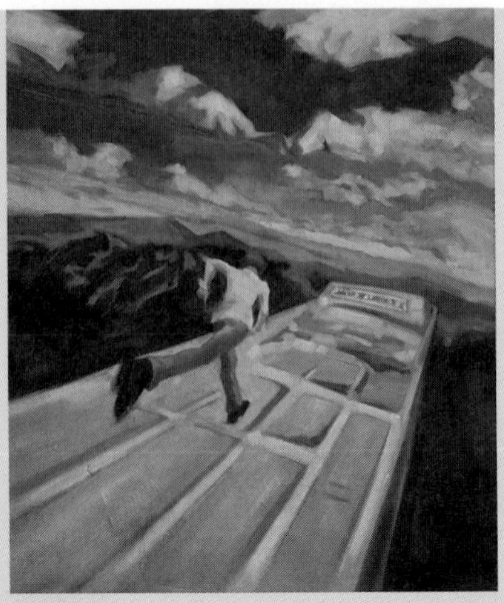

Milliequivalents

Learning Objectives

After completing this chapter, you should be able to:

- Explain the importance of electrolytes and milliequivalents in pharmacy.
- Calculate the needed volume of individual electrolytes.
- Calculate the total volume of electrolytes in a TPN.
- Determine the number of milliequivalents in a solution.
- Determine the number of milliequivalents in a dose.

INTRODUCTION

Electrolytes in solution conduct electricity. When electrolytes are dissolved in water, they split into charged particles known as ions, which carry an electric charge. Electrolytes are important in maintaining acid-base balance in body fluids, controlling body water volume, and regulating metabolism. Milliequivalents are used to express the concentration of electrolytes in solution.

Solutions can be isotonic, hypertonic, or hypotonic depending on their concentration as it relates to the osmotic pressure of human red blood cells.

Isotonic solutions: Solutions that have an osmotic pressure equal to that of cell contents. Normal saline, sodium chloride 0.9% solution, is considered isotonic with human red blood cells.

Hypertonic solutions: Solutions that have greater osmotic pressure than cell contents. Hypertonic solutions cause cells to dehydrate and shrink.

Hypotonic solutions: Solutions that have a lower osmotic pressure than cell contents. Hypotonic solutions cause cells to take on water and expand.

Total Parenteral Nutrition

Total parenteral nutrition, also called TPN, is a solution made to replenish many of the body's basic nutritional needs. It also contains necessary body fluids, vitamins, and lipids. In essence, it is everything the human body needs to sustain nutritional needs. This chapter will focus on the measurement of milliequivalents. The TPN is a good example for this measurement, as the essential electrolytes used are generally measured in milliequivalents.

Electrolyte Solutions

Electrolytes are commonly added to TPNs according to the needs of the patient as indicated by the physician on the order. *Parenteral* indicates that the solution is delivered into the bloodstream via IV infusion.

Following is a list of common electrolyte solutions that are readily available in vials for injection. The technician must determine how many milliliters will be extracted from the stock vial and injected into the TPN bag. Each item is extracted from the stock vial and injected into the TPN bag one at a time. TPNs are prepared in the clean room using aseptic technique.

EXAMPLE 9.1

Electrolyte	Stock Vial	Rx Order	How Many mL?
NaCl (sodium chloride)	4 mEq/mL	60 mEq	______________

Sodium chloride is salt the body needs.

Simply divide the ordered amount by the concentration noted on the stock vial of each ingredient:

$$\frac{60}{4} = 15$$

15 mL of NaCl are needed.

PRACTICE PROBLEMS 9.1

Determine the volume of electrolytes needed.

1.

Electrolyte	Stock Vial	Rx Order	How Many mL?
Na phosphate (sodium phosphate)	4 mEq/mL	34 mEq	______________

Sodium phosphate is a form of phosphorus, a naturally occurring substance that is important in every cell in the body. One of its functions is to aid the body in evacuation of the bowel.

2.

Electrolyte	Stock Vial	Rx Order	How Many mL?
Na acetate (sodium acetate)	2 mEq/mL	20 mEq	______________

Sodium acetate is a source of sodium ions; one of its function is to act as a diuretic.

3. **Electrolyte** | **Stock Vial** | **Rx Order** | **How Many mL?**

Electrolyte	Stock Vial	Rx Order	How Many mL?
$MgSO_4$ (magnesium sulfate)	4 mEq/mL	30 mEq	_______________

Magnesium is a naturally occurring mineral that is important for many systems in the body, especially the muscles and nerves. Magnesium sulfate also increases water in the intestines, which may induce defecation.

4.

Electrolyte	Stock Vial	Rx Order	How Many mL?
K acetate	2 mEq/mL	10 mEq	_______________

5.

Electrolyte	Stock Vial	Rx Order	How Many mL?
KCl (potassium chloride)	2 mEq/mL	40 mEq	_______________

Potassium is a mineral that is found naturally in foods and is necessary for many normal functions of the body, especially beating of the heart.

6.

Electrolyte	Stock Vial	Rx Order	How Many mL?
K phosphate (potassium phosphate)	4.4 mEq/mL	10 mEq	_______________

7.

Electrolyte	Stock Vial	Rx Order	How Many mL?
Ca gluconate (calcium gluconate)	0.465 mEq/mL	20 mEq	_______________

Calcium is a mineral that is found naturally in foods. Calcium is necessary for many normal functions of the body, especially bone formation and maintenance. Calcium can also bind to other minerals (such as phosphate) and aid in their removal from the body. **Calcium gluconate** is used to prevent and treat calcium deficiencies.

A TPN order will consist of a number of electrolytes, as shown in the following table. After calculating the needed volume per electrolyte, you can then add up each of the answers to determine the total volume of electrolytes in the TPN, as shown.

Electrolyte	Stock Vial	Rx Order	How Many mL?
NaCl	4 mEq/mL	60 mEq	_______________
Na phosphate	4 mEq/mL	34 mEq	_______________
K acetate	2 mEq/mL	20 mEq	_______________
$MgSO_4$	4 mEq/mL	30 mEq	_______________
Na acetate	2 mEq/mL	10 mEq	_______________
KCl	2 mEq/mL	40 mEq	_______________
K phosphate	4.4 mEq/mL	10 mEq	_______________
Ca gluconate	0.465 mEq/mL	20 mEq	_______________

Add the numbers in the last column to get the total volume of electrolytes: _______________

Other Calculations Involving Milliequivalents

You can calculate many problems regarding milliequivalents using simple ratios and proportions. Set up the ratio and proportion using the information given, place units appropriately, and then cross-multiply to solve.

Consider potassium chloride products, which are commonly prescribed.

$$\text{Molecular weight of KCl} = 74.5$$
$$\text{Equivalent weight of KCl} = 74.5$$
$$1 \text{ mEq of KCl} = 74.5 \text{ mg}$$

In the following examples, we will use these conversion values to calculate the number of milligrams provided in some common KCl products.

EXAMPLE 9.2 KCl 10 mEq

Set up the ratio and proportion:

$$\frac{1 \text{ mEq}}{74.5 \text{ mg}} :: \frac{10 \text{ mEq}}{x \text{ mg}}$$

Cross-multiply and solve for x:

$$x = 745 \text{ mg}$$

KCl 10 mEq contains 745 mg of potassium chloride. The accurate calculation is 745 mg; however, this is commonly rounded to 750 mg. Note also that manufactured products labeled as KCl 10 mEq contain 750 mg.

EXAMPLE 9.3 KCl 8 mEq

Set up the ratio and proportion:

$$\frac{1 \text{ mEq}}{74.5 \text{ mg}} :: \frac{8 \text{ mEq}}{x \text{ mg}}$$

Cross-multiply and solve for x:

$$x = 596 \text{ mg, commonly rounded to } 600 \text{ mg}$$

EXAMPLE 9.4 KCl 20 mEq

Set up the ratio and proportion:

$$\frac{1 \text{ mEq}}{74.5 \text{ mg}} :: \frac{20 \text{ mEq}}{x \text{ mg}}$$

Cross-multiply and solve for x:

$$x = 1490 \text{ mg, commonly rounded to } 1500 \text{ mg}$$

EXAMPLE 9.5 KCl 10% solution 480 mL

To determine the number of milliequivalents of KCl in this solution, you must first determine how many grams of KCl there are. Multiply the percentage of the solution, expressed as a decimal, by the total volume:

$$0.10 \times 480 = 48 \text{ g}$$

Once you have established the amount of KCl, set up the ratio and proportion. Do not forget to convert the weight of KCl in grams to milligrams—units must be the same when cross-multiplying:

$$\frac{1 \text{ mEq}}{74.5 \text{ mg}} :: \frac{x \text{ mEq}}{48{,}000 \text{ mg}}$$

Cross-multiply and solve for x.

$$x = 644 \text{ mEq}$$

EXAMPLE 9.6 Continuing with the solution given in Example 9.5, if the dose is 10 mL, then how many milliequivalents are in one dose?

Set up another ratio and proportion, cross-multiply, and solve for x:

$$\frac{644 \text{ mEq}}{480 \text{ mL}} :: \frac{x \text{ mEq}}{10 \text{ mL}}$$

$$x = 13.42 \text{ mEq per 10-mL dose}$$

How many milligrams of KCl are in the 10 mL dose?

Again, you will set up another ratio and proportion based on the information you have, cross-multiply, and solve for x:

$$\frac{1 \text{ mEq}}{74.5 \text{ mg}} :: \frac{13.42 \text{ mEq}}{x \text{ mg}}$$

$$x = 999.79 \text{ mg, rounded to 1000 mg, per 10-mL dose}$$

PRACTICE PROBLEMS 9.2

Solve the following milliequivalent-based problems.

KCl 20% Solution

The molecular weight of KCl = 74.5

The equivalent weight of KCL = 74.5

1 mEq of KCl = 74.5 mg

1. How many grams of KCl are in 100 mL of KCl 20% solution?

   ____

2. How many milliequivalents of KCl are in 100 mL of KCl 20% solution?

   ____

3. How many milliequivalents of KCl are in a 10-mL dose of KCl 20% solution? ______________

4. How many milligrams of KCl are in a 10-mL dose of KCl 20% solution?

   ____

SUMMARY

Milliequivalents are a specialized type of pharmacy calculation; most pharmacy technicians will not be required to calculate such problems due to either their practice setting or new automated technology. However, milliequivalents are still an important principle for all pharmacy professionals to be familiar with.

CHAPTER REVIEW QUESTIONS

MULTIPLE CHOICE

1. Sodium phosphate solution contains 96.4 mEq of sodium per 20 mL. How many milliequivalents of sodium are in a 30-mL dose? ______________
   a. 144.6 mEq c. 63.63 mEq
   b. 600 mEq d. 125 mEq
2. Milk of magnesia contains 80 mEq of magnesium per 30 mL. How many milliequivalents of magnesium are in 60 mL? ______________
   a. 144 mEq c. 180 mEq
   b. 160 mEq d. 240 mEq
3. Epsom salts contain 40 mEq of magnesium per 5 g. How many milliequivalents of magnesium are in a 5-lb. container? ______________
   a. 200 mEq c. 2500 mEq
   b. 454 mEq d. 18,160 mEq
4. How many mEq/mL are in sodium bicarbonate injection 7.5%? (molecular weight = 84, 1 mEq = 84 mg) ______________
   a. 0.9 mEq/mL c. 0.84 mEq/mL
   b. 0.6 mEq/mL d. 0.75 mEq/mL
5. How many grams of active ingredient are in 100 mL of KCl 20% solution? ______________
   a. 10 g c. 74.5 g
   b. 20 g d. 42 g
6. You have a stock vial of calcium gluconate injection 4.65 mEq/10 mL. How many milliliters do you need to provide 70 mEq? ______________
   a. 70 mL c. 150 mL
   b. 120 mL d. 325 mL
7. You have a stock vial of ammonium chloride 5 mEq/mL. How many milliliters do you need to provide a dose of 200 mEq? ______________
   a. 40 mL c. 80 mL
   b. 60 mL d. 100 mL
8. You have a stock vial of sodium bicarbonate 0.5 mEq/mL. How many milliliters do you need to provide 80 mEq? ______________
   a. 40 mL c. 120 mL
   b. 80 mL d. 160 mL
9. You have a stock vial of magnesium sulfate 4 mEq/mL. How many milliliters do you need to provide 24 mEq? ______________
   a. 4 mL c. 8 mL
   b. 6 mL d. 12 mL
10. How many milligrams of KCl 20% solution are in 1 mEq? ______________
    a. 0.0745 mg c. 7.45 mg
    b. 0.745 mg d. 74.5 mg

TRUE OR FALSE

11. Electrolytes in solution have charged particles called electrons. ______________
    a. true b. false
12. TPNs are administered through a nasogastric tube into the patient's gut. ______________
    a. true b. false
13. TPNs are prepared in the general compounding area of the pharmacy. ______________
    a. true b. false
14. You can determine the total volume of electrolytes in a preparation by adding together the volume of each electrolyte added to the solution. ______________
    a. true b. false

15. The molecular weight of an electrolyte equals 1 mEq of that electrolyte expressed in milligrams. (Example: KCl molecular weight = 74.5, therefore, 1 mEq = 74.5 mg)

____

a. true b. false

SHORT ANSWER

16. List three ways that electrolytes are useful in the body.

____

____

____

17. Describe how to calculate the volume of electrolytes needed for a preparation.

____

18. Describe how to determine the number of grams of electrolyte in a 10% electrolyte solution.

____

19. Show a calculation that proves there are 600 mg in 8 mEq of KCl.

____

20. Describe the series of steps used to determine how many milligrams per dose are in an electrolyte solution.

____

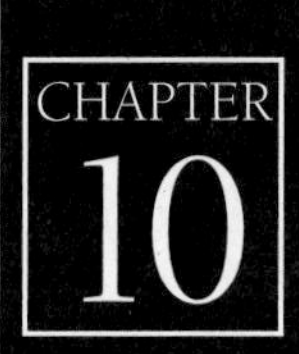

Basic Accounting and Operations

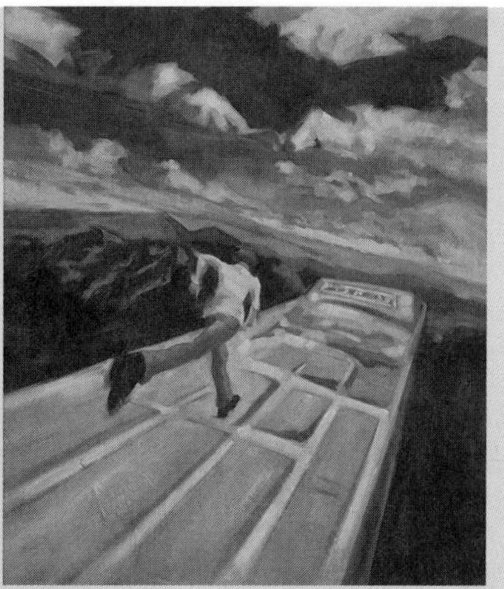

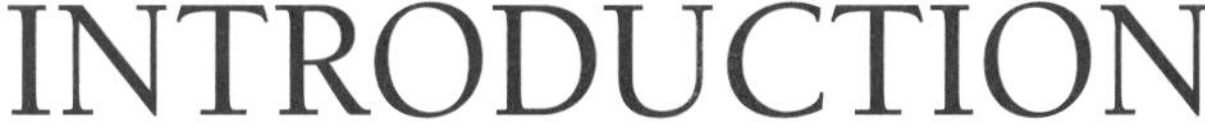

The goal of any business is to make a profit; pharmacy is no different. It is necessary to maintain enough profit in the business model to be able to take care of obligations such as rent and inventory expense and have a positive net income at the end of the fiscal year. Profits help pay salaries of employees, so it is important to keep a certain profit margin above supply costs so that the business can afford to keep and pay its employees.

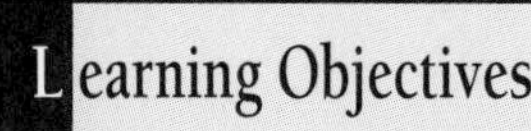

After completing this chapter, you should be able to:

- Define and understand how to calculate cost, selling price, and markup.
- Explain co-payments and AWP.
- Define and know how to determine markup and markup percent.
- Define and understand how to calculate gross profit and net profit.

Pharmacy Is a Business

In order to maintain a profitable business, many pharmacies have had to diversify their products and services. In addition to dispensing prescriptions, many pharmacies now offer immunizations, specialty compounds, nutritional counseling, and disease state management services. There is an art to managing a pharmacy in a way that cares for patients and the prices they pay for medicines while providing a business model that results in a positive net income. Controlling inventory, accounts receivable, cash flow, and variable expenses are all vital components of a successful business.

Accounting and Pricing Considerations

Cost: The amount the store paid for the drug, noted on the invoice and wholesaler sticker affixed to the stock bottle. Many pharmacies have set up a code in which each letter in the code represents a number. This invoice cost is then printed on the wholesaler sticker by using the code, or using numerals.

P H A R M O C I S T

1 2 3 4 5 6 7 8 9 0

The code shown here is not misspelled—there must be ten different letters for the code to properly work.

Cost is sometimes referred to as *invoice cost* or *acquisition cost*. Cost is used when taking quarterly or annual inventory.

Selling Price: The total amount to be paid for the product.

Over-the-Counter Products: The selling price for over-the-counter items is noted on the price sticker placed on the product or may be scanned by a bar code. When you ring up the customer, the selling price is the amount that you key or scan into the cash register. Wholesalers provide price stickers to be attached to each over-the-counter product. Some stores use bar-code scanning and show the price on a shelf tag.

Co-Payment: Many prescriptions are filled under third-party prescription plans for which the patient must pay a co-payment. Co-payments vary and may be a standard amount or a percentage of the total prescription price.

Tiered Co-Payments: Many third-party plans operate under a tiered co-payment system. For example, generic products might be $15.00, preferred brand-name products $30.00, and non-preferred brand-name products $50.00; some products may be excluded from coverage.

For prescription products, the total selling price includes the amount to be paid by the third-party insurer and the patient's co-payment. Reimbursement formulas set by the plan are used to calculate the total price for each prescription. Pharmacy computer systems communicate with the insurer through a computer data switch. Total price and the customer co-payment are transmitted back to the pharmacy system at the time of processing.

AWP: Average wholesale price. Most pharmacy systems perform a price update function weekly to update all drug files to the most current AWP data. This is critical because nearly all third-party plans use a pricing formula based on AWP—for example, AWP − 14% + $2.50.

Once the price is calculated according to the plan formula, the patient is responsible for the designated co-payment and the insurance company is responsible for the balance. The balance due to the pharmacy is batched with other claims from the same processor, and payment is transmitted to the pharmacy by check or electronic funds transfer along with a reconciliation statement. Many states have implemented prompt-payment legislation to help pharmacies collect payment in a timely manner. Some plans provide reconciliation statements through the Internet.

Markup: The difference between the selling price and the cost, stated in dollars and cents. You can calculate markup by using either of the following formulas:

$$\text{Selling price} - \text{Cost} = \text{Markup}$$

or

$$\text{Cost} + \text{Markup} = \text{Selling price}$$

Markup Percent: Use the following formula to calculate markup percent:

$$\frac{(\text{Selling Price} - \text{Cost})}{\text{Cost}} \times 100 = \text{Markup percent}$$

EXAMPLE 10.1 If an item that cost $70.00 is marked up to $100.00, what is the markup percent?

$$\frac{(100 - 70)}{70} \times 100 = 42.86\%$$

This can be verified: $70.00 × 1.4286 = $100.00

Overhead: Added costs needed to maintain the business. Overhead includes items such as electricity, rent, phone, and payroll. Cost of goods is not a part of overhead.

Gross Profit: When considering price and markup on prescription products, the industry uses the term *gross profit* to mean how much above cost the pharmacy is paid for a given prescription. This is calculated the same way as markup:

$$\text{Selling price} - \text{Invoice cost} = \text{Gross profit}$$

This tells us the gross profit for the particular prescription, but does not consider a number of other factors related to the cost of doing business.

Gross Profit Percent: This figure is calculated the same way as markup percent:

$$\frac{(\text{Price} - \text{Cost})}{\text{Cost}} \times 100 = \text{Gross profit percent}$$

Net Profit: Money left over after you pay invoice cost and overhead. Net profit is the last line found on a standard accounting income statement. A negative number reflects a net loss.

Income Statement: A simplified accounting income statement looks like this:

Income	100%	(all of the money that comes in)
– Cost of goods sold	70%	(cost for inventory purchases)
– Overhead and expenses	20%	(cost for overhead and salaries)
= Net profit	10%	(what's left over)

Let's compare two different income statements. Notice how much the net profit is improved when holding down expenses.

	Store #1		Store #2	
Income	$1,500,000	(100%)	$1,500,000	(100%)
– Cost of goods sold	$1,050,000	(70%)	$1,050,000	(70%)
– Overhead and expenses	$300,000	(20%)	$270,000	(18%)
= Net profit	$150,000	(10%)	$180,000	(12%)

Improving net profit by 2%, through either better purchasing or reducing expenses, resulted in an additional $30,000 per year. If purchases and expenses are minimized, the other way to increase net profit is through increased prices. This is difficult in today's market due to the large volume of third-party plans that have a contract formula for calculating selling price.

Many pharmacies have 80% or more of their volume tied to third-party plans. The cost of goods sold percentage shown, 70%, is a sample target. In today's market, very few stores actually achieve a 30% margin. However, average overhead and expenses for most businesses run around 18–20% of sales. This creates a strain on net profit. Therefore, pharmacies should be diligent in controlling inventory.

Inventory: All retail businesses must take an inventory at least annually, and some even do so quarterly. An inventory count is required at the end of the fiscal year and is necessary to accurately reflect the store's annual net profit. Inventory is taken at the cost of the product and is usually conducted by an outside firm.

Accounting Formulas

FORMULA **Selling Price**

$$\text{Selling price} = \text{Cost} + \text{Markup}$$

FORMULA **Markup**

$$\text{Markup} = \text{Selling price} - \text{Cost}$$

FORMULA **Markup Percent**

$$\text{Markup percent} = \frac{(\text{Selling price} - \text{Cost})}{\text{Cost}} \times 100$$

FORMULA **Gross Profit**

$$\text{Selling price} - \text{Invoice cost} = \text{Gross profit}$$

FORMULA **Gross Profit percent**

$$\frac{(\text{Price} - \text{Cost})}{\text{Cost}} \times 100 = \text{Gross profit percent}$$

FORMULA **Net Profit**

$$\text{Net profit} = \text{Selling price} - (\text{Cost} + \text{Overhead})$$

PRACTICE PROBLEMS 10.1

Perform the following pricing calculations.

1. If special-order items are marked up at 25% above AWP, what is the selling price for an item that has an AWP of $13.29?

   ____

2. If invoice cost of an item is $7.00 and the selling price is $13.89, how much is the markup? What is the markup percent? ______________

   ____

3. Advanced herbal and vitamin formulations are marked up 50% over invoice cost. If the invoice cost is $12.30, what is the selling price? How much is the markup? ______________ ______________

4. Hemorrhoid suppositories are priced at $3.29 and their invoice cost is $1.80. What is the amount of the markup? What is the markup percent? ________________ ________________

5. Weekly medication planners are marked up at 96% above invoice cost. A new display has arrived with an invoice and no suggested retail pricing stickers provided. What is the selling price for each item?
   a. 7-day pill pack, invoice cost $3.50 ________________
   b. 7-day pill pack with alarm, invoice cost $4.84 ________________
   c. 1-day pill box, invoice cost $0.64 ________________
   d. 28-day pill organizer tray, invoice cost $7.64 ________________

6. Glucometer test strips are sold for $98.00 per box of 100 strips. The net profit on the strips is $22.00. Store overhead per box of strips is $4.30. What is the invoice cost for the box of strips? ________________

7. High-protein nutrition drink packets have an invoice cost of $32.00 per box. The selling price is $52.95. Overhead is $3.90. What is the net profit for the item? ________________

8. Digital blood pressure monitors are priced at your pharmacy for $42.89 and the cost is $34.59. Overhead is 4% of cost. What is the net profit?

   ____

Use the following sample plan formulas to solve the following problems.

Brand-name product formula:	AWP − 14% + $2.50
Generic product formula:	AWP − 35% + $1.75

9. Product ABC has an invoice cost of 18.00/C. This means $18.00/100 capsules. The AWP is $36.30/C. The prescription calls for 42 capsules. ABC is a generic antibiotic.
   a. What is the selling price according to the plan formula?

      ____
   b. What is the gross profit? ________________
   c. What is the gross profit percent? ________________

10. Brand-name product XYZ nasal spray has an invoice cost of "PRSTT" using the cost code provided at the beginning of the chapter. The AWP for the product is $175.65.
    a. What is the selling price?________________
    b. What is the gross profit? ________________
    c. What is the gross profit percent? ________________

For each of the following price stickers, use the sample third-party formulas to calculate the selling price for 30 units, the gross profit, and the gross profit percent.

11. Accupril Sticker

    Cost: $97.05/90

    AWP: $122.31/90

    ________________ ________________ ________________

12. Xenical Sticker
    Cost: $108.01/100
    AWP: $132.86

    ______________ ______________ ______________

13. Diltiazem Sticker
    Cost: $63.00
    AWP: $130.10

    ______________ ______________ ______________

14. Tri-Sprintec Sticker
    Generic birth control
    7/7/7 pack
    Packaged 6 × 28
    Cost $140.02
    AWP: $218.68

    ______________ ______________ ______________

SUMMARY

As with all businesses, pharmacies must give special attention to accounting and operational calculations. Inventory mismanagement, improper pricing, and inadequate reimbursement can quickly cause a pharmacy to lose money.

CHAPTER REVIEW QUESTIONS

MULTIPLE CHOICE

1. What is the selling price for a product that costs $8.50 and has a 29% markup? ______
   a. $8.79 c. $17.00
   b. $10.97 d. $24.65
2. What is the markup percent for a product that costs $20.00 and sells for $39.95? ______
   a. 19.95% c. 50%
   b. 20% d. 99.75%
3. Which of the following is an example of overhead? ______
   a. payroll c. inventory
   b. markup d. cost of goods sold
4. Using the formula AWP − 14% + $2.50, what is the gross profit percent for 30 tablets of a product that has an AWP of $87.00/C and an invoice cost of $62.34/C? ______
   a. 18.70% c. 24.95%
   b. 33.41% d. 6.25%
5. Using the formula AWP − 35% + $2.50, what is the gross profit for 30 tablets of a generic product that has an acquisition cost of $42.60/C and an AWP of $164.35/C? ______
   a. $2.50 c. $21.77
   b. $12.78 d. $34.55
6. Determine the overhead for a product with a selling price of $89.00, cost of $62.00, and net profit of $8.50. ______
   a. $8.50 c. $28.50
   b. $18.50 d. $38.50
7. Determine the selling price for a product with a cost of $6.42, overhead of $1.89, and net profit of $2.00. ______
   a. $10.31 c. $1.89
   b. $6.42 d. $2.00
8. Determine the cost for a product with a selling price of $29.38, overhead of $4.50, and net profit of $8.00. ______
   a. $12.50 c. $24.88
   b. $21.38 d. $16.88
9. Determine the net profit for a product with a selling price of $68.49, cost of $42.00, and overhead of $7.50. ______
   a. $18.99 c. $49.50
   b. $34.50 d. $26.99
10. What is the markup percent for a product that costs $10.00 and sells for $13.99? ______
    a. 3.99% c. 10%
    b. 39.9% d. 13.9%

TRUE OR FALSE

11. Net profit can be improved by reducing expenses and increasing prices. ______
    a. true b. false
12. Controlling inventory expense is important to the profitability of the pharmacy. ______
    a. true b. false
13. Inventory should be conducted at least once a year. ______
    a. true b. false

14. The equation for net profit can be set up vertically and visualized as a simple accounting statement. ____________

    a. true b. false

15. The formula for markup percent is (Selling price − Cost)/Cost × 100.

    ____

    a. true b. false

SHORT ANSWER

16. Give an example of a tiered co-payment system.

    ____

17. Create a cost code that can be used to show product cost on a price sticker supplied by the wholesaler.

    ____

18. Describe markup and how it can be calculated.

    ____

19. List three items that are contained in overhead.

    __________ __________ __________

20. What is the formula for calculating net profit for individual products?

    ____

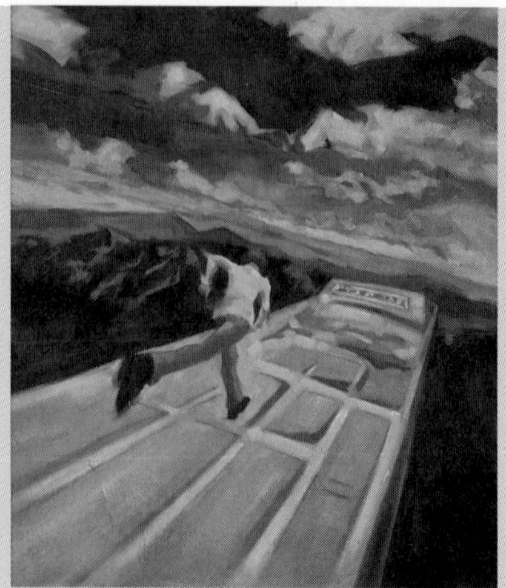

Practical Examples

This chapter contains a variety of practice problems. Expect to use all the different math principles discussed in the book.

1. Rx hydrocortisone 2.5% cream 240 g

   How many grams of active ingredient are in 240 g of cream?

   ____

2. Rx normal saline 1 L

   How many grams of sodium chloride are in 1 L of normal saline (NaCl 0.9%)? ________________

3. Rx 50 g of active ingredient in 1 L distilled water

   What is the percent strength of this product? ________________

4. Rx progesterone cream 100 mg/mL 60 mL

   a. What is the percent strength of this product? ________________

   b. How many grams of progesterone do you need to prepare the product? ________________

5. Rx 1:400 soaking solution 2 L

   What is the percent strength of the soaking solution?

   ____

6. Rx erythromycin 10% healing ointment 120 g

   How many grams of erythromycin should you use to prepare the order?

   ____

7. Rx sodium sulfacetamide 10% in lotion 90 mL

   How many grams of sodium sulfacetamide should you use to prepare the order? ________________

8. Rx urea 20% in betamethasone valerate crm 180 g

   How many grams of urea should you use to prepare the order?

   ____

9. How many milliliters are in 1 gal.? ______________

10. How many milliliters are in 1 L? ______________

11. How many milliliters are in 1 tsp? ______________

12. How many milliliters are in 1 Tbsp? ______________

13. How many pounds are in 1 kg? ______________

14. How many grams of drug are in 100 mL of a 10% solution?

    ____

15. How many grams of drug are in 100 g of a 20% cream?

    ____

16. How many grams of drug are in 30 g of a 1% ointment?

    ____

17. If a product contains 2 mg/5 mL and the dose is 1.5 tsp, how many milligrams of drug are in each dose? ______________

18. How many milliliters of dexamethasone 0.5 mg/5 mL are required to provide a dose of 2 mg? ______________

19. How many kilograms does a 165-lb. person weigh? ______________

20. How many kilograms does a 16-lb. canine weigh? ______________

21. How many kilograms does a 56-lb. child weigh? ______________

22. How many milligrams are in 1 gr? ______________

23. How many grains of codeine are in a tablet containing 300 mg acetaminophen and 60 mg of codeine? ______________

24. How many milligrams of nitroglycerin are in a tablet containing nitroglycerin 1/300 gr? ______________

25. How many milligrams would the dose be for a 56-lb. patient who is to take 7.5 mg/kg/day in four divided doses? ______________

26. How many milligrams would the dose be for a 140-lb. adult taking 20 mg/kg/day in one dose? ______________

27. How many milligrams would the dose be for a patient taking two KCl 10 mEq tablets daily? ______________

28. How much NaCl 4 mEq/mL stock solution is required to provide 20 mEq of NaCl? ______________

29. How many milligrams are in 10 g? ______________

30. How many grams are in 635 mg?______________

31. How many grams are in 1 gr? ______________

32. Dry-skin lotion has an invoice cost of $1.68 and sells for $2.49; what is the markup percent? ______________

33. Elastic bandage wraps have an invoice cost of $1.42 and sell for $2.89; what is the amount of the markup? ________________

34. Blood pressure monitors sell for $54.89, cost is $36.40, and net income is $14.49. What is the overhead? ________________

35. Vaporizers sell for $17.49, overhead is 4% of the selling price, and net income is $8.00 per unit. What is the cost? ________________

36. Convert 45° F to Celsius. ________________

37. Convert 98.6° F to Celsius. ________________

38. Convert −10° C to Fahrenheit. ________________

39. Convert 15° C to Fahrenheit. ________________

40. Rx Intron-A (interferon) 25 million U/5 mL
    a. What is the concentration in U/mL? ________________
    b. How many milliliters are required to provide a dose of 15 million U? ________________

41. Rx ciprofloxacin 200 mg/100 mL IVPB 100 mL over 60 min
    What is the flow rate in gtt./min? ________________

42. Rx vancomycin 1 g/200 mL IVPB 200 mL over 60 min
    The IV administration set delivers 20 gtt./mL. What is the flow rate in gtt./min? ________________

43. Rx morphine 10 mg/70 kg
    You have a stock vial of morphine 10 mg/mL. The patient weighs 200 lb. The IV bag holds 500 mL of D5W.
    a. What is the patient's weight in kilograms? ________________
    b. How many milligrams of morphine do you need to provide the recommended dose? ________________
    c. How many milliliters of stock solution will you need?
    d. What is the flow rate in gtt./min if the dose is given over 6 hr? ________________

44. Rx amphotericin-B 0.1 mg/mL 3 mg/kg/day over 4 hr
    Mix in D5W only.
    Protect from light.
    Refrigerate. Must be used within 24 hours.
    Flush line with D5W or use separate line.
    You have a stock vial of amphotericin-B 100 mg/50 mL. The patient weighs 265 lb. The IV administration set delivers 20 gtt./mL.
    a. What is the patient's weight in kilograms? ________________
    b. What is the recommended daily dose in milligrams? ________________
    c. How many milliliters of stock solution will you need? ________________
    d. What is the flow rate in gtt./min? ________________

45. Rx tobramycin 3 mg/kg/day q8h, 100 mL over 45 min

You have a stock vial of tobramycin 40 mg/mL. The patient weighs 140 lb. The IV administration set delivers 60 gtt./mL.

a. What is the patient's weight in kilograms? ________________

b. What is the recommended mg/dose? ________________

c. How many milliliters of tobramycin from the stock vial are needed?

____

46. Rx normal saline 1 L over 12 hr

What is the flow rate in gtt./min? ________________

47. Rx D5W 2 L over 22 hr

What is the flow rate in gtt./min? ________________

48. Rx TPN 1000 mL over 6 hr

What is the flow rate in gtt./min? ________________

49. Rx furosemide 80 mg over 2 min

You have a stock vial of furosemide 10 mg/mL.

a. How many mL/min will be supplied? ________________

b. How many mg/min will be injected? ________________

c. What is the flow rate in gtt./min? ________________

50. Rx nitroglycerin 25 mg/250 mL Infuse 250 mL

The recommended infusion rate is 50 mcg/1 min.

a. How many micrograms are in the 250-mL container?

____

b. How many hours will be required to administer the nitroglycerin?

____

c. What is the flow rate in gtt./min? ________________

51. Rx amikacin sulfate 500 mg 100 mL

What will be the infusion time if the IV administration set delivers 15 gtt./mL and is set at 30 gtt./min? ________________

52. Rx hydrocortisone 1.5% ointment 120 g

How many grams of hydrocortisone 2.5% ointment should you mix with white petrolatum to prepare the order? ________________

53. Rx betamethasone valerate 0.05% 240 g

How many grams of betamethasone valerate 0.1% should you mix with cream base to prepare the order? ________________

54. Rx povidone iodine 5% ointment

How many grams of povidone iodine 20% ointment should you mix with 45 g of povidone iodine 2% ointment to prepare the order?

____

55. Rx 10% soaking solution

How many milliliters of distilled water should you mix with 200 mL of a 50% stock solution to prepare the order? ________________

56. Rx acetic acid 0.25% 1 L

How many milliliters of stock solution of acetic acid 30% should you dilute to make the order? ________________

57. Rx cytarabine arabinoside 100 mg daily

How many milliliters of stock solution of cytarabine arabinoside 2 g in 20 mL will provide the required dose? ________________

58. Rx testosterone cypionate 25 mg/0.5mL 10 mL

How many milliliters of testosterone cypionate 200 mg/mL stock solution should you dilute to prepare the order? ________________

59. How many grams of product can you make by starting with 30 g of a 20% cream to make a 5% cream? ________________

60. How many milliliters of a 10% solution can you make by diluting 500 mL of a 25% stock solution? ________________

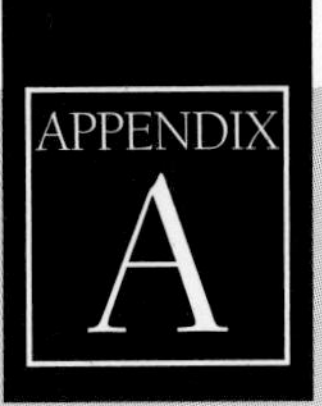

APPENDIX A

Answers

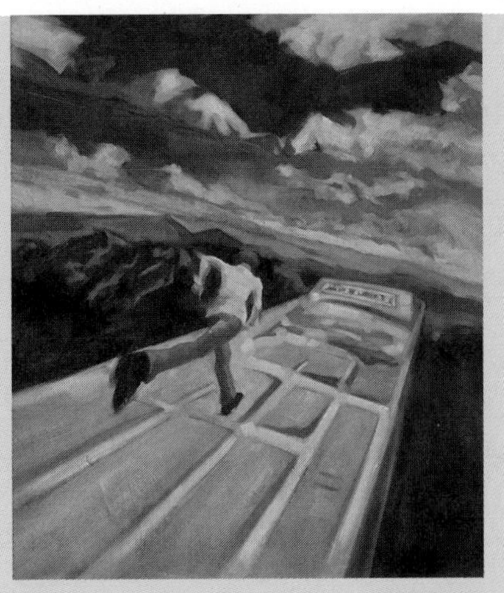

CHAPTER 1
Basic Math Overview

ANSWERS TO DIAGNOSTIC PRETEST:

1. 6.35
2. 1.89
3. 0.44
4. 40.0
5. 0.016
6. 7.01
7. 8.14
8. 64.115
9. 8.251
10. 8.935
11. 6.658
12. 16.53
13. 1.725
14. 6.2905
15. 17.05
16. 4.35
17. 14.667
18. 0.909
19. 10.7 oz.
20. $556.31
21. $9.78
22. 10
23. 1000
24. 50
25. 23
26. 2050
27. 47
28. $\frac{19}{24}$
29. $\frac{29}{45}$
30. $\frac{11}{21}$
31. $\frac{1}{24}$
32. $\frac{7}{8}$
33. $\frac{41}{56}$
34. $\frac{1}{15}$
35. $\frac{500}{3}$
36. $\frac{3}{80}$
37. $\frac{2}{3}$
38. $\frac{3}{5}$
39. $\frac{3}{14}$
40. 1310
41. 7680
42. $600
43. $x = 12$
44. $x = 2$
45. $x = 72$
46. 8%
47. 80%
48. $\frac{37}{100}$
49. 1:3
50. 1:500

PRACTICE PROBLEMS 1.1

1. 3.8
2. 6.05
3. 11.19
4. 10.4
5. 12.19
6. 0.11
7. 7.05
8. 0.1
9. 0.125
10. 0.06

PRACTICE PROBLEMS 1.2

1. 4.92
2. 3.22
3. 5.33
4. 864.656
5. 12.294
6. 399.99
7. 8.044
8. 64.194
9. 1.6976
10. 13.53

PRACTICE PROBLEMS 1.3

1. 2.545
2. 5.95
3. 9.09
4. 7.5
5. 6.11

PRACTICE PROBLEMS 1.4

1. 16.25
2. 5.45
3. 3.33
4. 8.75
5. 80

PRACTICE PROBLEMS 1.5

1. XCIV
2. CCCLXVII
3. XXVIII
4. MMDCL
5. CCCLXVIII
6. 39
7. 219
8. 898
9. 1,994
10. 49
11. 620
12. 1,331
13. 32
14. 34
15. 15

PRACTICE PROBLEMS 1.6

1. $\frac{13}{12}$ or $1\frac{1}{12}$
2. $\frac{17}{12}$ or $1\frac{5}{12}$
3. $\frac{127}{40}$ or $3\frac{7}{40}$
4. $\frac{3}{16}$
5. $3\frac{1}{4}$
6. $\frac{3}{10}$
7. $\frac{5}{32}$
8. $\frac{5}{12}$
9. $\frac{4}{5}$
10. $\frac{21}{20}$ or $1\frac{1}{20}$
11. $\frac{1}{2}$
12. $\frac{21}{2}$ or $10\frac{1}{2}$

ANSWERS TO CHAPTER REVIEW QUESTIONS

1. 4.1
3. 0.8
5. 3.7
7. 4.8
9. 12.01
11. 13.24
13. 6.80
15. 2.5
17. XXV
19. LXVII
21. 24
23. 86
25. 78
27. $5\frac{1}{5}$
29. $\frac{1}{2}$
31. $\frac{5}{12}$
33. $\frac{1}{75}$
35. $\frac{3}{20}$
37. 24
39. $1\frac{6}{7}$
41. 3 mg
43. 8.75 mg
45. 1965
47. $1\frac{7}{24}$ oz.
49. 16 mL

CHAPTER 2
Systems of Measurement

PRACTICE PROBLEMS 2.1

1. 5 mcg
2. 0.2 mg
3. 16 g
4. 0.05 kg
5. 10 mL
6. 3.1 L
7. 0.2 mcg
8. 500 mg
9. 0.06 g
10. 100 mL
11. 41 L
12. 0.7 mcg
13. 0.08 mg
14. 2000 g
15. 4.1 mL
16. 350 L
17. 7.4 g
18. 1000 mcg
19. 1500 mg
20. $1\frac{1}{5}$ kg
21. 0.025 mg
22. 0.1 g
23. 0.0006 kg
24. 1500 g
25. 220 mg
26. 1,500,000 mcg
27. 1 mg
28. 15,600 mL
29. 1.5 L
30. 200,800,000 mcg
31. 0.56632 L
32. 0.988 g
33. 12.5 mg
34. 7.5 L
35. 789 mL
36. 0.0001 g
37. 6000 kg
38. 105,000 mL
39. 2,000,000,000 mcg
40. 1000 mL

PRACTICE PROBLEMS 2.2

1. 2.8 kg
2. 12 tablets
3. a. 500 mg
   b. 500 mg
4. 692.322 g
5. 3.75 g
6. 36 bottles
7. 0.85 g
8. 212.5 mg
9. 1173.7 g
10. five tablets

PRACTICE PROBLEMS 2.3

1. 20 units
2. 10,000 units
3. 1,000,000 units
4. 53 units
5. 200,000 units
6. 2300 units
7. 100 units
8. 1000 units
9. 60 units
10. 700 units

PRACTICE PROBLEMS 2.4

1. 50 mEq
2. 30 mEq
3. 40 mEq
4. 5 mEq
5. 15 mEq
6. 20 mEq
7. 80 mEq
8. 100 mEq
9. 10 mEq
10. 55 mEq

PRACTICE PROBLEMS 2.5

1. 50 mEq
2. 10 tsp
3. 15 oz.
4. 10 Tbsp
5. 100 U
6. 7 gtt.
7. 2 pt.
8. 6 qt.
9. 3 gal.
10. 500 U
11. 10 gr
12. $\frac{1}{2}$ oz.
13. 16 pt.
14. $2\frac{1}{2}$ gr
15. 30 oz.

ANSWERS TO CHAPTER REVIEW QUESTIONS

1. d
3. a
5. f
7. e
9. m
11. n
13. l
15. a. true
17. b. false
19. a. true
21. the metric, apothecary, and household systems
23. the number of grams of a drug in 1 mL of a normal solution

CHAPTER 3
Conversions of Measurement

PRACTICE PROBLEMS 3.1

1. 15 mL
2. 1920 mL
3. 15 mL
4. 90 mL
5. 11,520 mL
6. 1.6 tsp
7. 3360 mL
8. 2270 g
9. 4.9 pt.
10. 1350 mL
11. 36 pt.
12. 1.5 oz.
13. 132 lb.
14. 4 tsp
15. 180 mL
16. 6 pt.
17. 40 oz.
18. 6 qt.
19. 1.5 cups
20. 96 tsp
21. 1.6 tsp
22. 96 tsp
23. 42 vials
24. 404 Tbsp
25. 96 tsp

PRACTICE PROBLEMS 3.2

1. 325 mg
2. 5 drams
3. 975 mg
4. 113.6 g
5. 9.2 gr
6. 15 mL
7. 0.88 oz.
8. 19.8 lb.
9. 10.8 mg
10. 10 drams
11. 8 oz.
12. 3250 mg
13. 7.7 lb.
14. 7.5 oz.
15. 2400 oz.
16. 1.5 lb.
17. 45 kg
18. 32.5 mg
19. 4.6 gr
20. 4 mL
21. 40.9 mg
22. 5 oz.
23. 7.3 kg
24. 13 mg
25. 65 mg every eight hours
26. 1.25 tablets
27. 180 mL
28. 0.8 oz.
29. 1.5 g
30. 48 mL

PRACTICE PROBLEMS 3.3

1. 15° C
2. 37.2° C
3. 37.8° C
4. 26.7° C
5. 54.4° C
6. 39.2° F
7. 89.6° F
8. 66.2° F
9. 101.1° F
10. 50° F
11. 46.1° C
12. 36° to 37.8° C
13. 98.6° F
14. 37.8° C
15. 13.3° C

ANSWERS TO CHAPTER REVIEW QUESTIONS

1. a. 1.8 lb.
3. b. 10 pt.
5. d. −16.7° C
7. d. 101 lb.
9. c. 0.18 g
11. a. true
13. b. false
15. a. true
17. In the apothecary system 1 lb. = 12 oz., but in the household system 1 lb. = 16 oz.
19. four days

CHAPTER 4
Ratios and Proportions

PRACTICE PROBLEMS 4.1

1. $\frac{2}{4}$, reduces to $\frac{1}{2}$
2. $\frac{6}{8}$, reduces to $\frac{3}{4}$
3. $\frac{1}{25}$
4. $\frac{1}{400}$

PRACTICE PROBLEMS 4.2

1. 4:5
2. 9:10
3. 1:400
4. 1:20

PRACTICE PROBLEMS 4.3

1. $\frac{4}{5} \times 100 = 80\%$
2. $\frac{9}{13} \times 100 = 69.23\%$
3. $\frac{1}{25} \times 100 = 4\%$
4. $\frac{1}{200} \times 100 = 0.5\%$
5. $\frac{1}{50} \times 100 = 2\%$
6. $\frac{1}{400} \times 100 = 0.25\%$
7. $\frac{1}{10} \times 100 = 10\%$
8. $\frac{4}{16} \times 100 = 25\%$
9. 25 g/100 mL
10. 1.25 g/100 g
11. 0.05 g/100 g
12. 0.04 g/100 mL

PRACTICE PROBLEMS 4.4

1. $x = 7$
2. $x = 3495$

ANSWERS TO CHAPTER REVIEW QUESTIONS

1. a. $\frac{1}{6}$
3. d. 12.5%
5. b. 2.5 g
7. c. 900
9. a. 1.5
11. a. true
13. a. true
15. a. true
17. Identify the diagonal that does not contain x and multiply those numbers. Next, identify the diagonal that contains x and divide by the number shown on that diagonal.
19. Restate the ratio as a fraction, then multiply by 100. (Example: 1:4, $\frac{1}{4} \times 100 = 25\%$)

CHAPTER 5
Dosage Calculations

PRACTICE PROBLEMS 5.1

1. Convert 0.05% to a decimal:
   $0.0005 \times 3.5 = 0.00175$ g
2. 12.5 mg
3. Convert 0.12% to a decimal:
   $0.0012 \times 15 = 0.018$ g. Then convert grams to milligrams by moving the decimal point three places to the right: 18 mg.
4. a. 40 doses b. 10 days
5. 10 mg
6. a. 225 mg of estriol and 75 mg of estradiol
   b. 0.9375 mg of estriol and 0.3125 mg of estradiol; the total dose is 1.25 mg.
   Note that the dose indicated is 0.5 g of a product that is 2.5 mg/g: $\frac{2.5}{2} \times 0.75 = 0.9375$ of estriol, $\frac{2.5}{2} \times 0.25 = 0.3125$ of estradiol.

7. a. 50 doses b. 0.25 g
8. a. 18 tablets b. 9 days
9. 0.461 gr. (Note: this would commonly be rounded to 0.5 gr in practice.)
10. 8.33 mL

PRACTICE PROBLEM 5.2

Fried's Rule

$$\text{Child's dosage} = \frac{\text{Age in months}}{150} \times \text{Adult dosage}$$

$$\frac{24}{150} \times 650 = \frac{15{,}600}{150} = 104 \text{ mg Tylenol}$$

$$\frac{24}{150} \times 500 = \frac{12{,}000}{150} = 80 \text{ mg amoxicillin}$$

Young's Rule

$$\text{Child's dosage} = \frac{\text{Age of child in years}}{\text{Age of child in years} + 12} \times \text{Adult dosage}$$

$$\frac{2}{2 + 12} \times 650 = \frac{1300}{14} = 93 \text{ mg Tylenol}$$

$$\frac{2}{2 + 12} \times 500 = \frac{1000}{14} = 71 \text{ mg amoxicillin}$$

Clark's Rule

$$\text{Child's dosage} = \frac{\text{Weight in pounds}}{150} \times \text{Adult dosage}$$

$$\frac{22}{150} \times 650 = \frac{14{,}300}{150} = 95 \text{ mg Tylenol}$$

$$\frac{22}{150} \times 500 = \frac{11{,}000}{150} = 73 \text{ mg amoxicillin}$$

PRACTICE PROBLEMS 5.3

1. a. 40 kg b. 1000 mg c. 250 mg
2. a. 30.9 kg b. 1390 mg c. 695 mg
3. a. 10 kg b. 10 mg
4. a. 28.18 kg b. 5.64 mg c. 1.88 mg
5. a. 24.5 kg b. 150 mg (the order states not to exceed 150 mg) c. 75 mg

ANSWERS TO CHAPTER REVIEW QUESTIONS

1. b. 64 doses
3. c. 80 mL
5. b. 48 days
7. a. 10 mg
9. a. 2.5 mg
11. a. true
13. b. false
15. a. true
17. ointments, syrups, tablets
19. 2 mg

CHAPTER 6
Concentrations and Dilutions

PRACTICE PROBLEMS 6.1

1. 2.5% w/w
2. 1.25% w/w
3. 5% w/v
4. 10% v/v

PRACTICE PROBLEMS 6.2

1. 4 mL
2. 2880 mL
3. 250 mL (Note: Remember to state the concentrations in percent strength.)
4. 1:3333 (Note: The final percent strength of the soaking solution is 0.03%.

   Restate 0.03% as a fraction: $\frac{0.03}{100}$.

   Next divide 0.03 into 100: $\frac{100}{0.03} = 3333$.

   Therefore, the ratio is 1:3333.)

---

5. 0.4 mL
6. 120 mL
7. 83.33 mL
8. 7.5 mL
9. 2.4 mL
10. 15 mL
11. 0.3 mL
12. 10 mL

PRACTICE PROBLEMS 6.3

1. 5 g
2. 1.2 g
3. a. 30 doses b. 30 tablets
4. 2.25 g

ANSWERS TO CHAPTER REVIEW QUESTIONS

1. a. 50 g
3. b. 0.01%
5. d. 30 mL
7. c. 2.4%
9. b. 1.2 g
11. b. false
13. a. true
15. a. true
17. With % w/w, the final product is a solid such as a cream or ointment; with % w/v, the final product is a liquid such as a syrup or suspension.
19. The diluent is the larger volume that is mixed with the stock solution or active ingredient.

CHAPTER 7
Alligations

PRACTICE PROBLEMS 7.1

1. 250 mL of the 1% solution and 750 mL of water
2. 250 mL of the 4% solution and 750 mL of water
3. 45 g of the 10% ointment and 75 g of the 2% ointment
4. 1.33%
5. 5%
6. 1:50
7. 1:3.03
8. 1:4
9. 8.33 mL
10. 7.5 g
11. 5055 mL
12. 12 g
13. 75 mL
14. 15 g of the 20% ointment and 30 g of the 5% ointment
15. 192 mL
16. 0.01 mL
17. 37.5 g

ANSWERS TO CHAPTER REVIEW QUESTIONS

1. c. 4.88 g
3. c. 25 g of the 10% cream and 95 g of the 0.5% cream
5. d. 12.6 g
7. a. 1:2
9. b. 12 g
11. a. true
13. a. true
15. b. false
17. a. Express the strengths as a percent when setting up the problem.
    b. Always use a leading zero when writing percents or using decimals.
    c. Water, vanishing cream base, and petrolatum are considered a percent strength of zero.
19. Rewrite the ratio strength as a fraction and multiply by 100.

CHAPTER 8
Flow Rates

PRACTICE PROBLEMS 8.1

1. a. 500 mg b. 33.3 min
2. a. 500 mg b. 67 gtt./min c. 67 mL/hr
3. a. 86 kg b. 21,500,000 U/day c. 42 mL/hr d. 833,333 U/hr
4. a. 6.36 kg b. 1.59 mg c. 0.4 mL d. 100 gtt./min
5. 7.94 hr
6. 1440 mL
7. 4.17 hr
8. a. 31 gtt./min b. 125 mL/hr
9. a. 0.833 hr b. 40 mg/min c. 20 mg/mL
10. a. 50 gtt./min b. 0.67 U/min

ANSWERS TO CHAPTER REVIEW QUESTIONS

1. d. 67 mg/min
3. a. 27 gtt./min
5. b. 50 gtt./min
7. a. 5 mL
9. c. 10 mL
11. a. true
13. a. true
15. a. true
17. mL/hr × gtt./mL × 1hr/60 min = gtt./min
19. 60 gtt./mL

Chapter 9
Milliequivalents

PRACTICE PROBLEMS 9.1

1. 8.5 mL
2. 10 mL
3. 7.5 mL
4. 5 mL
5. 20 mL
6. 2.27 mL
7. 43.01 mL

PRACTICE PROBLEMS 9.2

1. 20 g
2. 268.5 mEq
3. 26.85 mEq
4. 2000 mg

ANSWERS TO CHAPTER REVIEW QUESTIONS

1. a. 144.6 mEq
3. b. 18,160 mEq
5. b. 20 g
7. a. 40 mL
9. b. 6 mL
11. b. false
13. b. false
15. a. true
17. Divide the ordered amount by the concentration noted on the stock vial.
19. 1 mEq/74.5 mg :: 8 mEq/x mg

    Cross multiply. $x = 596$ mg, this is commonly rounded to 600 mg.

Chapter 10
Basic Accounting and Operations

PRACTICE PROBLEMS 10.1

1. $16.61
2. $6.89, 98.4%
3. $18.45, $6.15
4. $1.49, 82.7%
5. a. $6.86 b. $9.49 c. $1.25 d. $14.97
6. $71.70
7. $17.05
8. $6.92
9. a. $11.66 b. $4.10 c. 54.23%
10. a. $153.56 b. $4.56 c. 3%
11. $37.56, $5.21, 16.10%
12. $36.77, $4.37, 13.49%
13. $27.12, $8.22, 43.5%
14. $25.44, $2.11, 9.04%

ANSWERS TO CHAPTER REVIEW QUESTIONS

1. b. $10.97
3. a. payroll
5. c. $21.77
7. a. $10.31
9. a. $18.99
11. a. true
13. a. true
15. a. true
17. Each letter of the code represents a number; there must be 10 different letters in the code.

    F A M I L Y D R U G

    1 2 3 4 5 6 7 8 9 0
19. Rent, utilities, payroll.

Chapter 11
Practical Examples

1. 6 g
2. 9 g
3. 5%
4. a. 10% b. 6 g
5. 0.25%
6. 12 g
7. 9 g
8. 36 g
9. 3840 mL
10. 1000 mL
11. 5 mL
12. 15 mL
13. 2.2 pounds
14. 10 g
15. 20 g
16. 0.3 g
17. 3 mg
18. 20 mL
19. 75 kg
20. 7.27 kg

21. 25.45 kg
22. 65 mg
23. 1 gr
24. 0.216 mg
25. 47.72 mg
26. 1272.8 mg
27. 1490 mg
28. 5 mL
29. 10,000 mg
30. 0.635 g
31. 0.065 g
32. 48.2%
33. $1.47
34. $4.00

---

35. $8.79
36. 7.22 degrees Celsius
37. 37 degrees Celsius
38. 14 degrees Fahrenheit
39. 59 degrees Fahrenheit
40. a. 5,000,000 U/mL b. 3 mL
41. 100 gtt./min
42. 67 gtt./min
43. a. 90.9 kg b. 12.98 mg c. 1.3 mL
    d. 83 gtt./min
44. a. 120.45 kg b. 361 mg c. 180.5 mL
    d. 15 gtt./min
45. a. 63.64 kg b. 63.64 mg/dose
    c. 1.6 mL
46. 83.33 gtt./min
47. 90.90 gtt./min
48. 167 gtt./min
49. a. 4 mL/min b. 40 mg/min
    c. 240 gtt./min
50. a. 25,000 mcg b. 8.33 hours
    c. 30 gtt./min

---

51. 50 minutes
52. 72 g
53. 120 g
54. 9 g
55. 800 mL
56. 8.33 mL
57. 1 mL
58. 2.5 mL
59. 120 g
60. 1250 mL

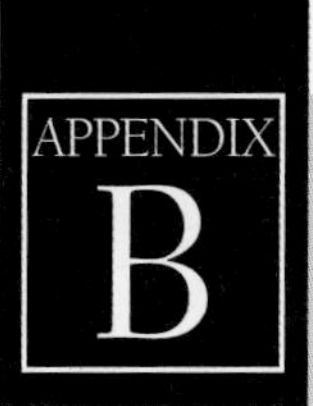

Resources and References

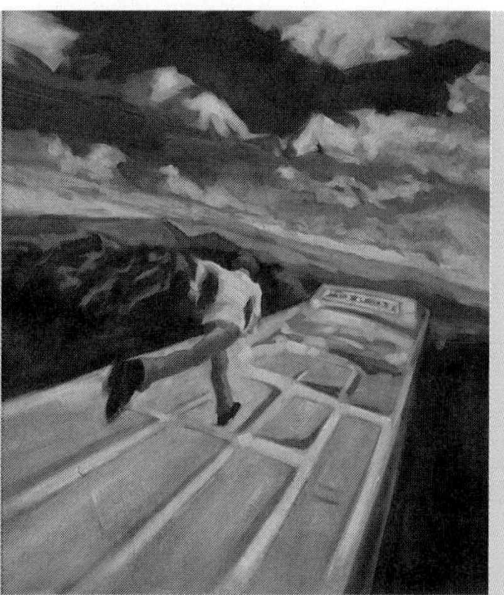

Ansel, Howard C., and Mitchell J. Stoklosa. *Pharmaceutical Calculations*, 11th ed. Philadelphia, Pa.: Lippincott, Williams & Wilkins, 2001.

"A Brief History of Measurement Systems." October 2004. **http://www.slcc.edu/schools/hum_sci/physics/tutor/2210/measurements/history.html**.

Facts and Comparisons. *Drug Facts and Comparisons*. St. Louis, Mo.: FC, 1998.

Hopkins, William A., Jr. *APhA's Complete MATH Review for the Pharmacy Technician*. Washington, DC: American Pharmaceutical Association, 2001.

Kocher, Keith. *Pharmacy Certified Technician Calculations Workbook*. Lansing: Michigan Pharmacists Association, 1994.

Miller, Dianne E., and Franz Neubrecht. *Pharmacy Certified Technician Calculations Workbook*. Lansing: Michigan Pharmacists Association, 2003.

The Pharmacy Technician. Englewood, CO: Morton, 1999.

Remington's Pharmaceutical Sciences, 16th ed. Easton, Pa.: Mack, 1980.

Index

G

H

I

K

L

M

N

O

P